CARDIAC SURGERY

Current Issues 1

CARDIAC SURGERY

Current Issues 1

Edited by

Aurel C. Cernaianu

and

Anthony J. DelRossi

University of Medicine and Dentistry of New Jersey
Robert Wood Johnson Medical School at Camden
Camden, New Jersey

SPTINGER SCIENCE+BUSINESS MEDIA, LLC

Library of Congress Cataloging in Publication Data

Cardiac surgery: current issues / edited by Aurel C. Cernaianu and Anthony J. Del-Rossi.
p. cm.
Includes bibliographical references and index.
ISBN 978-0-306-44319-0 ISBN 978-1-4615-3418-1 (eBook)
DOI 10.1007/978-1-4615-3418-1
1. Heart—Surgery—Congresses. 2. Heart—Surgery—Nursing—Congresses. I. Cernaianu, Aurel C. II. DelRossi, Anthony J.
[DNLM: 1. Heart Surgery—congresses. WG 169 C26725]
RD598.C346 1992
617.4'12059—dc20
DNLM/DLC 92-49455
for Library of Congress CIP

Proceedings of a symposium entitled Cardiac Surgery: 1992,
held November 7-10, 1991, in St. Thomas, U.S. Virgin Islands

ISBN 978-0-306-44319-0

Originally published by Plenum Press, New York in 1992

PREFACE

This monograph is intended to compile the lectures presented at the 4th Annual Symposium "Cardiac Surgery:1992" held at the Frenchman's Reef Beach Resort, St. Thomas, US Virgin Islands, November 7-10, 1991. This symposium was organized by the Division of Cardiothoracic Surgery and the School of Cardiovascular Perfusion, Cooper Hospital/University Medical Center, Camden, New Jersey and sponsored by the University of Medicine and Dentistry of New Jersey, Robert Wood Johnson Medical School at Camden, Philadelphia Academy of Cardiovascular Perfusion and the American Society of Extracorporeal Technology - Region II.

The symposium was devoted to cardiothoracic surgeons, cardiologists, cardiovascular perfusionists, and nurses involved in the management of the cardiac surgical patient. Therefore, the context of the book represents the multidisciplinary nature of cardiac surgery at its present level of development.

The contributors to this book have critically examined their experience and discussed controversial issues regarding cardiac pathophysiology, surgical indications, operative techniques, and long-term care and outcome.

The co-editors wish to express their gratitude for the contributors' efforts in the production of this manuscript. We would also like to thank the members of the Organizing Committee, Jane V. Stewart MSN, RN, CCRN, Roger A. Vertrees BA, CCP, Rosemary Volosin, MSN, RN, Rosemary Morrone and Paul R. Cappola BS, CCP, who have greatly contributed to the success of the symposium.

We would also like to express our thanks for the valuable support and assistance provided by the exhibitors and sponsors of the symposium, and Ms. Mary Safford and the staff at Plenum Publishing Corporation.

Aurel C. Cernaianu, M.D. FICS

Anthony J. DelRossi, M.D. FACS

July 1992

COURSE DIRECTOR

Anthony J. DelRossi, M.D.
Chairman, Department of Surgery
Head, Division of Cardiothoracic Surgery
Cooper Hospital/University Medical Center
Associate Professor of Surgery
University of Medicine and Dentistry of New Jersey
Robert Wood Johnson Medical School at Camden
Camden, NJ

ORGANIZING COMMITTEE

Jane V. Stewart, MSN, RN, CCRN
Nurse Manager, Coronary Care Unit
Presbyterian University Medical Center
Philadelphia, PA

Rosemary Volosin, MSN, RN
Clinical Nurse Specialist
Division of Cardiothoracic Surgery
Cooper Hospital/University Medical Center
Camden, NJ

Roger A. Vertrees, BA, CCP
Program Director
School of Cardiovascular Perfusion
Cooper Hospital/University Medical Center
Camden, NJ

Paul R. Cappola, BS, CCP
President, AMSECT Region II
President, Philadelphia Academy of Cardiovascular Perfusion
Director, Cardiovascular Perfusion
Miriam Hospital
Providence, RI

Rosemary Morrone
Program Coordinator
Division of Cardiothoracic Surgery
Cooper Hospital/University Medical Center
Camden, NJ

EXHIBITORS

Avecor Cardiovascular, Inc. - Plymouth, MN
Baxter, Bentley Laboratories Division - Irvine, CA
BFW - Lexington, KT
Cobe Laboratories - Arcada, CO
Datascope Corporation - Montvale, NJ
Deknatel, Inc. - Fall River, MA
Electromedics, Inc. - Inglewood, CA
Ethicon, Inc. - Somerville, NJ
W. L. Gore and Associates, Inc. - Elkton, MD
IMPRA - Tempe, AZ
Luxtec Corporation - Sturbridge, MA
Mallinckrodt Sensor Systems, Inc. - Ann Arbor, MI
Medtronic, Inc. - Heart Valves - Minneapolis, MN
Medtronic, Inc. - Cardiopulmonary Division - Anaheim, CA
Hoffman LaRoche Laboratories - Nutley, NJ
St. Jude Cardiac Assist - Shelmsford, MA
St. Jude Medical, Inc. - St. Paul, MN
Sarns/3M Health Care - Ann Arbor, MI

SPONSORS

We are grateful for the generous financial support received from the following:

Abbott Laboratories, Hospital Products Division, Abbott Park, IL
Bard Cardiopulmonary - Tewksbury, MA
Glaxo Pharmaceuticals - Research Triangle Park, NC
Minntech Corporation - Minneapolis, MN
Shiley, Inc. - Irvine, CA
State of the Art Medical Products, Inc. - Rahway, NJ

CONTENTS

Mitral Valve Surgery 1
James R. Pluth

Myocardial Augmentation Using Skeletal Muscle 9
Robert Fietsam, Jr. and Larry W. Stevenson

Thoracic Transplantation 33
G. Michael Deeb, Steven F. Bolling, Edward L. Bove, Louis A. Brunsting, F. Mark Lupinetti and Mark B. Orringer

Coronary Bypass Grafting in Conjunction with Carotid and Valvular Disease 43
Anthony J. DelRossi and Aurel C. Cernaianu

Cardiac Anesthesia and Oxygen Delivery and Uptake in the Critically Ill 63
T. James Gallagher

Complex Cardiac Surgery 71
Denton A. Cooley

Cardiac Surgery Without Transfusion: A Reappraisal 91
Richard K. Spence

Physiology of Blood Flow During Cardiopulmonary Perfusion . . 101
Roger A. Vertrees and Louis Brownstein

Postoperative Responses to Hypothermia: Nursing Considerations 117
Jill A. Fikkert

Cardiac Valve Replacement in the 1990's: The Nursing Perspective 127
Susan Kiley Eckert

Intraoperative Care of the CABG Patient: A Nursing Diagnosis Approach 137
Gail Kaempf

ECMO: An Overview for Perfusionists 145
Mark Kurusz

Biomaterials and the Development of Membrane Technology . . . 161
Jeffrey P. Sites

The Physiologic Impact of Cardiac Surgery: The Nursing Perspective 175
Bonnie R. Sakallaris

The Automatic Implantable Cardioverter Defibrillator; Surgical Considerations and Pre- and Postoperative Nursing Care . 183
Rosemary Volosin

Thoracic Trauma and the Rupture of the Diaphragm 189
Joan Perks

Nursing Research: The Key to Excellence in Nursing Practice . . 197
Elizabeth H. Winslow

Contributors 203

Index 207

MITRAL VALVE SURGERY

James R. Pluth, M.D.

Mayo Clinic Scottsdale
Scottsdale, Arizona

Today, there are a multitude of prosthetic valves available for mitral valve replacement. These can generally be divided into bioprosthetics and mechanical valves. Of the mechanical valves, the Starr-Edwards valve has been employed since the early 1960's, and the current valve model has not changed or been modified since 1966 (Fig. 1a). Valve failure since that period of time is virtually unheard of, and the valve remains the gold standard against which durability can be compared. This valve has an unfavorable internal diameter-to-external diameter ratio, especially in the small sizes, as we will later discuss, and, therefore, may contribute to unfavorable gradients. The other class of mechanical valves are the tilting disc varieties. These include the St. Jude (Figure 1b), the Omni-Science (Figure 1c), the Medtronic-Hall (Figure 1d), and the Duramedic valve among others. The majority of these valves had their inception between 1977 and 1981, and all incorporate the use of ferropyrolite to reduce thromboembolic incidents and decrease valve wear. An infrequent complication of tilting disc valves, and one that usually occurs in the presence of inadequate coagulation, is valve thrombosis. This process is due to defibrinogenation of the blood, and the incidence is probably proportional to the number of struts through which blood must pass.

Of the bioprosthetic prostheses, the Hancock (Figure 2a), and Carpentier-Edwards (Figure 2b) are the most popular varieties. The Ionescu-Shiley pericardial valve is no longer available, but recently a low-profile Carpentier-Edwards pericardial valve has been introduced.

With this multitude of valves available, is there one prosthesis that is superior to the others in valve performance and makes it the logical choice for valve replacement? In the early years of valve surgery, McGoon[1] established a set of criteria against which valves could be compared. These criteria included durability, hemodynamic characteristics, thromboembolism, assurance of function, availability, choice of

Cardiac Surgery: Current Issues, Edited by A.C. Cernaianu
and A.J. DelRossi Plenum Press, New York, 1992

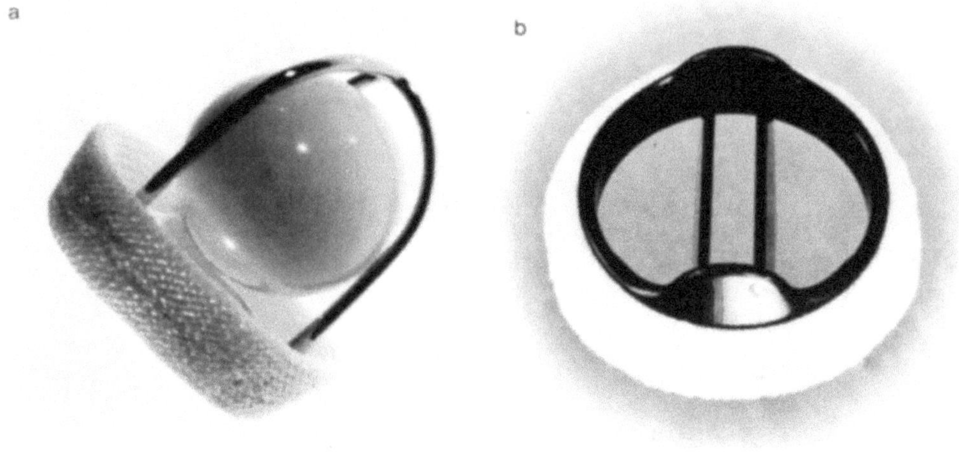

Figure 1. (a and b)

size, ease of insertion, and record of survival. Today, when choosing a mitral valve substitute, the availability, size, and ease of insertion should be considered. It is the remaining four criteria which constitute a source of comparison.

Bioprostheses have been characterized by early calcification and valve failures, especially in the younger age groups. In children, failure rates of 50 percent at five years have been reported,[2] and the rate appears to diminish as age advances. Etiology of early valve failure appeared to be related to increased calcium turnover rates which occurs in the younger individuals and in patients with renal failure or hyperparathyroidism. Generally, it is advisable to avoid using bioprosthetics in these categories of patients; however, the durability of this valve in

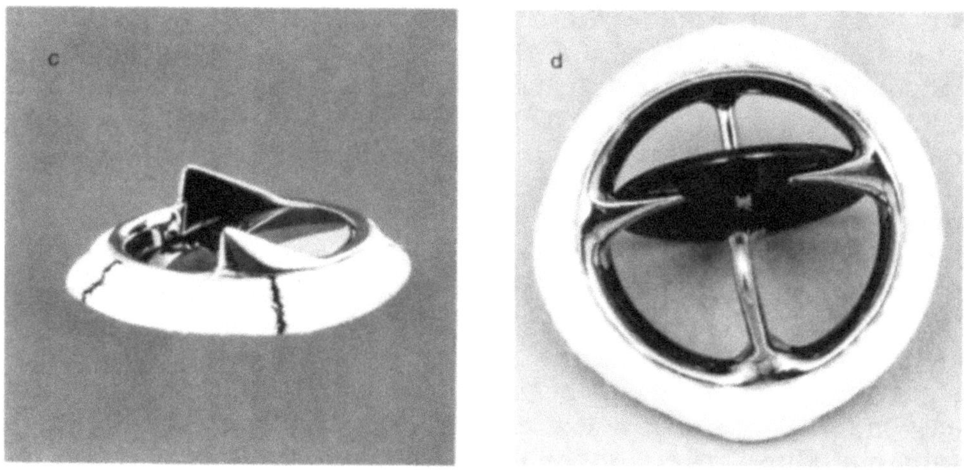

Figure 1. (c and d)

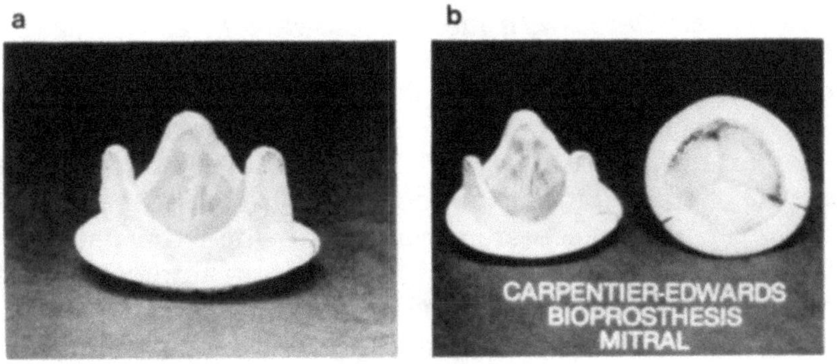

Figure 2. (a and b)

patients greater than 70 years of age is good, with about a 2 percent failure rate per year in the mitral position.[3]

Thromboembolic complications vary among valve types. In general, the thromboembolic complications are higher with mechanical valves than with bioprostheses. Among the mechanical valves, the ball-and-cage valve has the highest incidence of thromboembolic complications.[4] Generally, the risk for thromboembolism and anticoagulant complications for mechanical valves range between 4 and 8 percent per 100 patient years which, over a period of ten years, could be projected to be nearly a 60 percent risk. In contrast, the bioprosthetics have a risk of 2 to 3 percent per year, or about one-half that of the mechanical valve.

Hemodynamic differences do exist among valve types. The ball-and-cage valve has the most unfavorable inlet orifice area-to-valve mounting area. The tilting disc valves have slightly better performance data than the natural occurring bioprosthesis. With the exception of the Starr-Edwards valve, all mechanical and bioprosthetic valves 27 mm or greater in size have acceptable *stenotic gradients*. The *stenotic gradient* is only a part of the hemodynamic picture with prosthetic valves, the other aspect being that of regurgitation. In contrast to the aortic position where regurgitation occurs, both with valve closure, and for mechanical valves, throughout diastole, regurgitation in the mitral position occurs only during valve closure, and the duration of systole. The amount of regurgitation in the mitral position is, therefore, considerably less, being in the range of 6 to 8 percent of forward flow which is virtually insignificant. For bioprosthetics, regurgitant fraction is similar to the human valve at about 2 to 3 percent of forward flow. There is, therefore, no significant difference in left ventricular volume work due to the factor of regurgitation.

Survival appears to be a poor criterion for choosing a valve, since irrespective of which valve has been employed, the survival is generally the same.[5] About 75 percent of patients are alive at five years. Since all valves have inherent problems which are unique to their own design, the early failure rate and requirement for reoperation and bioprosthesis balances out the risk of thromboembolism and anticoagulant complications associated with mechanical valves.

With these factors in mind, is there an important difference in selecting a valve for a particular patient? In the mitral position, the criteria for this selection is mainly related to: (1) age; and (2) annulus size. If the patient is greater than 70 years of age, a bioprosthesis appears very acceptable. If the patient is younger, then consideration should be given to a mechanical valve, provided the patient will responsibly take anticoagulation, and has no contraindication to the use of anticoagulation. Because of the teratogenic effects of coumadin therapy, an argument could be made for the employment of bioprostheses in women of child-bearing age who are in sinus rhythm. Here, the individual must understand and accept the fact that valve replacement at the very first indication of valve failure will be required. Coronary artery surgery may influence the conduct of an operation in a patient requiring valve replacement. Generally, if a mechanical valve is being employed in a younger patient, all efforts should be made to revascularize with arterial type conduits to decrease the need for further surgery.

Annulus size is of secondary importance in mechanical valve replacement. With a small annulus, consideration should be given towards tilting disc valves which have more acceptable gradients than their bioprosthetic counterparts, and considerably improved function over the ball-and-cage valve.[6] The final decision in choice of valve is usually related to patient and physician choice, if all other factors are equal. Here, if one weighs the facts, the only logical conclusion is to opt not for valve replacement, but for valve repair, if this is feasible.[7]

Survivorship is significantly better with valve repair, being approximately 85 percent at five years despite the occasional need for reoperation. The difference between survivorship with valve repair versus replacement may well relate to the preservation of the left ventricular contraction mechanism that occurs with valve repair. When one excises the leaflets and the attached chordae, one can expect a 16 percent reduction in ventricular function from posterior leaflet division with an additional 25 percent reduction from anterior leaflet excision.[8] If one compares total excision of the mitral apparatus to preservation of the posterior leaflet and valve replacement, and compares these with valve repair, there is a progressive improvement in ejection fraction, decrease in left ventricular end-diastolic pressure, and proportionate increase in cardiac index. The difference in survivorship between repair and replacement has been noted by many authors, and does not appear to be influenced by the type of valve employed.[9] Additionally, valve repair is associated with a lower incidence of thromboembolic complications, and anticoagulation is not required in patients with a sinus mechanism.

How does one determine if valve repair can be accomplished? Basically, 90 percent of pure mitral regurgitation can be corrected by valve reparative procedures. Virtually, all the patients in whom regurgitation stems from the posterior leaflet, can be repaired. To determine whether valve repair is feasible, the best diagnostic tool remains that of simple auscultation. Posterior leaflet disruption presents as a holosystolic murmur audible mainly in the aortic valve area where, except for the shape and timing of the murmur, could well be confused with aortic stenosis. Anterior leaflet disruptions, in contrast, radiate to the spine, and even to the top of the skull by bony conduction. Murmurs which seem to originate from the rheumatic process with a fish-mouth orifice, are most audible in the axilla. In our experience, auscultation of the murmur has been more reliable than echocardiography in determining the source of regurgitation. Knowledge of the origin of the murmur is important since if repair cannot be accomplished, surgery should be offered at an earlier stage of the disease when the patient presents only with class II New York Heart Association (NYHA) symptomatology.

Careful assessment of the valve at the time of surgery is an essential first step. One must determine whether either one or both of the leaflets rise above the level of the annulus or if there is shortening of the leaflet with restrictive motion. If there is an overshoot deformity of one of the leaflets, one then needs to inspect the chordal mechanism to determine whether ruptured chordae, papillary muscle disruption, or simple elongation of the chordae is present. The most common pathology for pure mitral regurgitation is ruptured tendineae. When this condition is noted, numerous methods for repair are available. The McGoon repair[10] excludes the tea-spout deformity that results from disruption of the primary chordae. Generally, this excluded segment of valve is plicated beneath the valve toward the left ventricle presenting a smooth surface to the left atrium. The advantage of this method is that, in case of failure occurring from disruption of the suture repair, no increase in regurgitation is likely to develop. The disadvantage is that this traction from the repair can form a V-shaped deformity in the area of congenital clefts of the posterior leaflet, so that these must additionally be closed. Additionally, if there is a limited amount of leaflet tissue, central regurgitation can occur, although this can be offset with an annuloplasty. The Merindino repair[11] is similar to the McGoon repair with the exception that the excluded segment is excised. Similar disadvantages to the McGoon repair exist. In addition, increased regurgitation resulting from suture dehiscence may occur. The Carpentier repair[12] employs a quadrangular excision with concomitant decrease in annulus size at the time of reconstruction. The advantage of this procedure is that the anatomy of the valve is better maintained, although with disruption, an increase in regurgitation will occur. The repair is virtually always performed with an annuloplasty to reduce stress on the annulus. All of these methods are applicable to the posterior leaflet, but may be employed on the anterior leaflet if only 15 to 20 percent of the leaflet is involved.

When the chordae are intact but simply elongated, a shortening procedure can be effective in the repair. Here, the papillary muscle is cut, a loop of suture is placed around the redundant chordae, and the chordae drawn into the incised papillary muscle. There are a few reports currently in the literature reporting disruption of the chordae after this repair.[13] It is important that the suture be placed so that it is buried into the incision of the muscle, and subsequent healing is primarily between the chordae and the papillary muscle.

Chordal substitution can be employed both on anterior and posterior leaflets. Originally, Kay[14] suggested the procedure employing Tefdek® sutures as chordae substitutes. Subsequently, rolled glutaraldehyde-preserved pericardium has been utilized, and more recently, 5-0 Goretex suture has been suggested. When anterior leaflet disruption occurs, one can excise a rectangular segment of the posterior leaflet with the intact chordae, and suture them to the underside of the flailed anterior leaflet. The posterior leaflet can then be repaired as in the Carpentier repair.

With papillary muscle disruption, the tip of the papillary muscle can be reattached to the free wall of the left ventricle by suturing the segment into an incision in the endocardium at the appropriate distance from the annulus. The procedure is considerably easier to perform when associate aneurysmectomy is required, but under both circumstances, judging the appropriate distance from the annulus is a difficult process, and this judgment must be made when normal tension of the myocardium exists. In the presence of a relaxed heart from cardioplegia, overcorrection may occur with resultant displacement of the valve leaflets below the annulus plane when coronary perfusion is re-established.

In the presence of a dilated annulus, or with certain valvuloplasty repairs, an annuloplasty is often required. It appears to be prudent to employ an annuloplasty whenever a portion of the valve is excised in the process of repair, and is additionally required in about one-half the cases of the McGoon type repair when inadequate leaflet tissue is present. Whether utilizing a rigid or flexible ring, is somewhat a matter of debate, although contraction of the heart may be less impaired with a malleable ring.

Other methods of valve repair include the use of pericardial patch for healed subacute bacterial endocarditis (SBE) perforations. This patch does not require preserved pericardium unless a very large patch is being employed.

Results of valve repair are generally excellent, though at least with plication techniques, posterior repairs appear to fare better than anterior repairs. We cannot forget that the earliest procedure for valve repairs is that of commissurotomy. Today our colleagues in cardiology have virtually stolen from us this very rewarding procedure by employing balloon disruption of the valve.[16] The arguments in surgery regarding open or closed commissurotomy have long been debated. Advantage to the closed technique includes a lower morbidity, decreased cost which is important in Third World countries, and a lower incidence of valve replacement.[17] In contrast, proponents for the open method believe that it offers a more precise procedure with a potential for longer palliation and correction of subchordal narrowing. With current teaching, it is unusual for the newer surgeons to have experience with the closed method of repair so that the trend today is towards the open technique.

The advantages of valvuloplasty become obvious when survivorship is compared, especially with varying degrees of ejection fraction. In Kay's report, survivorship is not significantly different when the ejection fraction was greater than 40%. However, with values between 20 and 40 percent, marked differences in survivorship occurred, especially in dealing with patients with ejection fractions below 20%. Additionally, embolic-free survivorship is markedly improved with valve repair.

The major disadvantage with valve reparative procedures is that reoperation is occasionally required. The incidence of this is approximately 2 to 2.5 percent per year, and is markedly less with posterior plication repairs than those involving the anterior leaflet. It is of interest, however, that the risk of valve reoperation is not significantly higher in patients undergoing valve reparative procedures compared to those undergoing valve replacement.

REFERENCES

1. J.R. Pluth, D.C. McGoon: Current status of heart valve replacement. *Modern Concepts of Cardiovascular Disease* 43:65-70;1974.
2. D.B. Williams, G.K. Danielson, D.C. McGoon, F.J. Puga, D.D. Mair, W.D. Edwards: Porcine heterograft valve replacement in children. J Thorac *Cardiovas Surg* 84:446-450;1982.
3. E.L. Jones: Personal communication.
4. L.H. Edmunds, Jr: Thrombotic and bleeding complications of prosthetic heart valves. *Ann Thorac Surg* 44:430-445;1987.
5. D.A. Barnhorst, H.A. Oxman, D.C. Connolly, J.R. Pluth, G.K. Danielson, B. Wallace, D.C. McGoon: Long-term follow-up of isolated replacement of the aortic or mitral valve with the Starr-Edwards prosthesis. *Am J Cardiol* 35:228-233;1975.
6. D. Morse, R.B. Steiner, J. Fernandez (eds), Springer-Verlag, New York, *Guide to Prosthetic Cardiac Valves* 1985.
7. D.C. McGoon, (ed), F.A. Davis, Philadelphia, *Cardiac Surgery, edition 2*, 1987.
8. G.E. Sarris, D.C. Miller: Valvular-ventricular interaction: The importance of the mitral chordae tendineae in terms of global left ventricular systolic function. *J Cardiol Surg* 3:215-234;1988.
9. T.E. David: Mitral valve replacement with preservation of chordae tendinae: Rationale and technical considerations. *Ann Thorac Surg* 41:680-82;1986.
10. D.C. McGoon: Repair of mitral insufficiency due to ruptured chordae tendinae. *J Thorac Cardiovasc Surg* 39:357;1960.
11. K.A. Merendino, G.I. Thomas, J.E. Jesseph, et al: The open correction of rheumatic mitral regurgitation and/or stenosis. *Ann Surg* 150:5;1959.
12. A. Carpentier, S. Chauward, J.N. Fabiani, et al: Reconstructive surgery of mitral valve incompetence. *J Thorac Cardiovasc Surg* 79:338;1980.

13. Koutlas, et al: Chordal rupture as a late complication after mitral valve reconstruction. *J Thorac Cardiovasc Surg* 102:466-468;1991. (Letter)
14. J.H. Kay, W.S. Egerton: The repair of mitral insufficiency associated with ruptured chordae tendineae. *Ann Surg* 157:315;1963.
15. T.E. David: Replacement of chordae tendineae with expanded polytetrafluoroethylene sutures. *J Card Surg* 4:286-90;1989.
16. Multicenter experience with balloon mitral commissurotomy. NHLBI Balloon Valvuloplasty Registry Report on Immediate and 30-day Follow-up Results. The National Heart, Lung, and Blood Institute Balloon Valvuloplasty Registry Participants. *Circulation* 85:448-461;1992.
17. Balloon valvuloplasty versus closed commissurotomy for pliable mitral stenosis: A prospective hemodynamic study. *J Am Coll Cardiol* 18:1318-1322;1991.

MYOCARDIAL AUGMENTATION USING SKELETAL MUSCLE

Robert Fietsam, Jr., M.D. and Larry W. Stephenson, M.D.

The Department of Surgery
Division of Cardiothoracic Surgery
Wayne State University/School of Medicine
Detroit, Michigan

The development of intractable congestive heart failure occurs in nearly 400,000 people annually,[1,2] and has a 35% one year mortality.[3] An estimated 35,000 people per year could benefit from cardiac transplantation, yet less than 2000 donor hearts are available annually.[4] In the remaining 33,000 patients there is a 50% one year mortality rate.[5] For these patients, the alternative is an artificial heart, an intra-aortic balloon pump, or different variations of ventricular assist devices, however at this point these devices are temporary. Furthermore, they require percutaneous tubes or wires for transmission of energy from an external power source. Although experiments with a totally implantable assist device are planned for 1992,[6] problems with coagulopathy, strokes and infection still need to be solved.

Another alternative for the augmentation of cardiac function is the use of autogenous skeletal muscle. This has the advantage of being a readily available power supply without the potential for rejection. The contractile power of skeletal muscle can support the heart primarily in two ways. Cardiomyoplasty involves wrapping the latissimus dorsi muscle around the heart and stimulating it to contract synchronously during systole. This has been used clinically in an estimated 150 patients worldwide, including Argentina,[7] Brazil,[8,9] Canada, France,[10,11] USA,[12,13] and the USSR,[14,15] and is currently in stage II clinical testing by the FDA in this country.

The other method is the creation of a separate pumping chamber made of skeletal muscle. These pumping chambers or skeletal muscle ventricles (SMV) generate power at a level between that of the right and left ventricle and have performed well in animal models for up to 2.3 years.[16]

Cardiac Surgery: Current Issues, Edited by A.C. Cernaianu
and A.J. DelRossi Plenum Press, New York, 1992

HISTORY

Skeletal muscle was first used in heart surgery six decades ago. In 1931, a penetrating cardiac injury was repaired by De Jesus in Bolivia using pectoralis muscle.[17] Two years later, Leriche and Fontaine[18] published experimental work using a free autograft of pectoralis muscle to reinforce the myocardial scar of an infarcted canine heart. Experiments of Beck[19,20] and O'Shaughnessy[21] demonstrated that pedicle-muscle grafts placed on the heart developed vascular anastomoses between the two tissues, particularly if the myocardium was rendered ischemic. Beck used this procedure in 20 patients and documented a reduction of angina pectoris.[22,23] Petrovsky used the hemidiaphragm to obliterate and flatten left ventricular aneurysms in 100 patients.[24-29] The pectoralis and intercostal muscle have also been used for aneurysm repair.[30,31]

Kantrowitz was the first to attempt to use the contractile power of skeletal muscle to augment cardiac function.[34,33] He used two different methods. Pedicle grafts of the left hemidiaphragm were wrapped around the canine heart and stimulated to contract synchronously with the heart. Secondly, the canine hemidiaphragm was wrapped around the descending aorta and stimulated during diastole. They were not able to detect hemodynamic improvements with the first method. The second method produced a 26% increase in diastolic aortic pressure until the muscle fatigued after fifteen seconds. Later experiments with cardiomyoplasty on an ischemic heart showed increased left ventricular pressure, peak femoral artery pressure, and aortic blood flow.[34] Using synchronous stimulation with every other systole this effect lasted 3 hours, however with a 1 to 1 stimulation pattern, no hemodynamic improvement was noted after 15 minutes because of muscle fatigue. Similar short term effects were noted by Nakamura in 1964.[35]

Other muscles have been used in an attempt to support the heart, including the pectoralis, psoas, and the rectus abdominis.[36] The latissimus dorsi was used for cardiomyoplasty in 1966 by Termet[37] and by Hume in 1968.[38] Termet placed the muscle on the heart and eight months later, while fibrillating the heart, stimulated the thoracodorsal nerve to cause muscle contraction which he claimed produced a peak aortic pressure of 80 mmHg. He reported that he could maintain this pressure in the fibrillating heart for 15 minutes until the muscle fatigued.

Spotnitz designed a separate muscle pump from canine rectus abdominis muscle, which developed pressures up to 500 mmHg[39] but required a filling pressure of 150 mmHg and, as with the early work with cardiomyoplasty, the muscle fatigued rapidly. In 1977, von Recum made separate muscle pumping chambers using the diaphragm which also failed after several hours due to fatigue.[40]

Although cardiac augmentation as measured by increased aortic blood pressure, flow or augmented diastolic pressure was reported in these early experiments, the effect was always short lived due to the onset of muscle fatigue. The successful adaption of skeletal muscle for long term cardiac augmentation required the creation of a more fatigue resistant muscle.

BASIC MUSCLE RESEARCH

Skeletal muscle and myocardium both convert chemical energy into mechanical work. Their cellular ultrastructure is similar, having longitudinally arranged myofibrils, a transverse tubular system, and a sarcoplasmic reticulum within the contractile unit called a sarcomere.[41] The functional requirements of the two types of muscles are different and accordingly they have some different cellular characteristics. The myocardium works continuously, has 30% mitochondria by volume, and uses an aerobic metabolism. The cardiac muscle has a uniform myosin composition which uses energy more efficiently than skeletal muscle myosin and can achieve a maximum active tension of 0.5 kg/cm^2 of cross sectional area. Intercalated disks between cells function as low resistance pathways to allow current to flow easily from cell to cell, which allows the cardiac fibers to be stimulated simultaneously, in an "all-or-none" fashion, in response to a single electrical stimulation.

Skeletal muscle is composed of two types of cell fibers associated with two different myosin isotypes, "slow" and "fast". The slow-twitch, type I, fibers are more similar to cardiac cells, in that energy is obtained from aerobic, oxidative phosphorylation. This form of metabolism renders the cell relatively fatigue resistant. Fast-twitch, type II fibers, primarily use an anaerobic, glycolytic metabolism, have a larger sarcoplasmic reticulum and a smaller mitochondrial volume, and subsequently utilize their energy stores quickly, and fatigue readily.

Overall, skeletal muscle cells have only 2-5% mitochondria by volume but can generate a maximum active tension of 1-5 kg/cm^2 of cross sectional area. Unlike cardiac cells, skeletal muscle cells are organized into motor units with individual nerve endings, which enable the individual motor units to be stimulated independently. A succession of appropriately timed stimuli result in a summation of individual muscle contractions which augments force and duration of contraction.[36,42-49]

In 1960, working with cats, Buller, et al, switched the motor nerve of a muscle with predominantly type I fibers with the motor nerve of a muscle with predominantly type II fibers.[50,51] After neuron regeneration, the previously slow twitch muscle, the soleus, had a faster contraction rate, and the previously fast twitch muscle, the flexor digitorum longus, had an decreased contraction rate. In 1969, Salmons and Vrbova showed that it was the pattern of motor nerve stimulation that determined the muscle fiber type. They were able to convert a fast-twitch muscle to a slow-twitch muscle by mimicking the stimulation pattern normally delivered by the nerve of a slow twitch muscle using

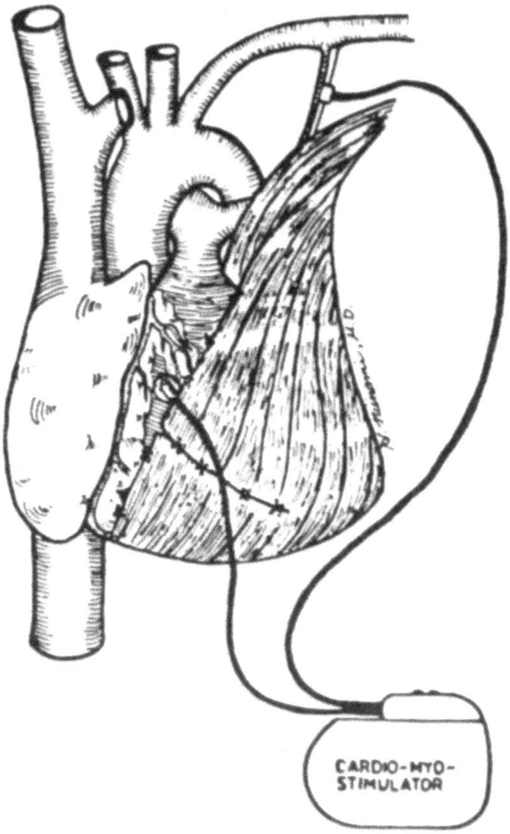

Figure 1a. Cardiomyoplasty with left latissimus dorsi muscle. Note the cardiac sensing lead and the stimulation lead to the thoracodorsal nerve. Others weave the nerve lead among the nerve fibers as the nerve enters the latissimus dorsi muscle.

an implanted nerve stimulator.[52] Salmons also showed increased fatigue resistance with long term stimulation.[53] Subsequent investigation revealed that chronic electrical stimulation changes the biochemical, morphologic, and physiologic characteristics of the muscle.[54-56] Studies in man have also shown an increased ratio of slow to fast twitch muscle types after eight weeks of endurance training.[57]

In the first week of electrical stimulation of the motor nerve, there is an increase in capillary density[56,58,59] followed by an increased mitochondrial volume concentration. Further stimulation results in a transformation of myosin isotype.[55,56] Increased activity of enzymes involved in oxidative phosphorylation and decreased activity of anaerobic pathway enzymes occurs.[60] This change highlights the importance of aerobic metabolism in the fatigue-resistant transformed muscle.[61] Hudlicka has shown increased activity of fatty acid activating enzyme and increased uptake of free fatty acids.[62] Studies of chronically stimulated canine skeletal muscle have shown that the alteration of anaerobic and aerobic metabolism is stable after two months of stimulation. However, enzymes involved in fatty acid catabolism and ketone body

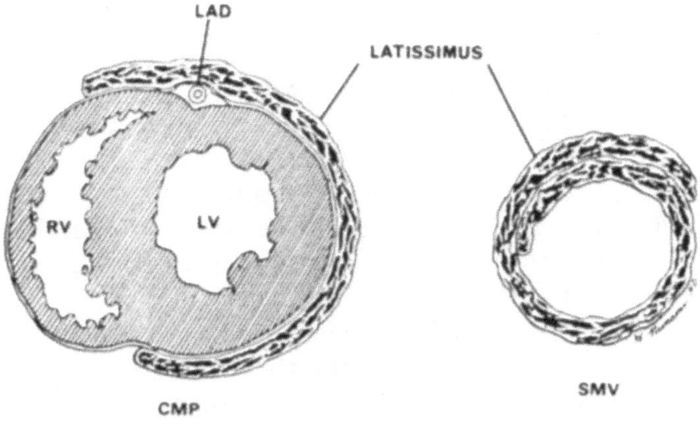

Figure 1b. Drawing of cross-sectional representation of cardiomyoplasty (CMP) and skeletal muscle ventricle (SMV). LV, left ventricle. RV, right ventricle. LAD, left anterior descending coronary artery.

catabolism show maximal activity after six months and remain significantly elevated after one year.[63] Furthermore, the lipid droplet volume fraction increases by 350% suggesting that chronically conditioned canine muscle uses fat as a main source of energy.

Electrical stimulation causes a change in the contractility of skeletal muscle during the first two weeks of conditioning. The relaxation time increases secondary to decreased activity of calcium-adenosine triphosphatase (ATPase) with a reduction of calcium ion binding and uptake in the sarcoplasmic reticulum membrane.[64,65] The isometric twitch contraction time decreases because of a change in calcium-binding proteins.[66]

Measurements of oxygen consumption show more efficient oxygen use by conditioned muscle.[67] Measurements of energy substrates with phosphorus-31-nuclear magnetic resonance during exercise tests also show that conditioned muscles have an increased capacity for oxidative phosphorylation which rivals the heart.[68] Multiple studies have confirmed the conversion of skeletal muscle to exclusively type I fiber using 2 Hz stimulation for 6 to 12 weeks.[40,52,53,56,69-72] Histochemical and physiologic studies of the canine latissimus dorsi after electrical stimulation for one year revealed no evidence of fiber damage, no abnormality of nerve conduction time, and no loss of acquired fatigue resistance.[73] Fiber size decreases initially while the percentage of nonmuscle tissue increases.[63] After one year of stimulation, comparing 120 to 54 contractions/min, the higher rate developed a lower isometric tension.[73] When stimulated at a rate similar to the intrinsic rate of the heart, transformed skeletal muscle loses less than 20% of its initial force with time.[1]

It seemed that it might be possible to exploit this phenomenon of muscle transformation for skeletal muscle cardiac assistance.[69,71,74]

Currently, the latissimus dorsi muscle is the preferred muscle for cardiomyoplasty. It has the advantage of a single main blood supply and motor nerve, it can be freed easily from its native position, is close to the heart, and it has a relatively large surface area which can cover up to 80% of the ventricular surface[75,76] (Figure 1). For the patient, its loss causes relatively little physical impairment because other muscles compensate for its function.[77] In addition, the muscle has a bulk comparable with that of the left ventricle,[48] and since skeletal muscle is capable of more work per unit weight then cardiac muscle[78] a single latissimus dorsi has the potential for assuming a major portion of the left ventricular workload. During mobilization of the latissimus dorsi from the chest wall, the collateral blood vessels to the muscle from the chest wall must be divided. The distal half of the muscle becomes ischemic. A three week vascular delay period allows recovery of normal resting and exercise-induced blood flow.[48,79,80]

Experimental work with latissimus dorsi cardiomyoplasty has shown inconsistent results. Chachques, et al, showed an increased right ventricle pressure in only one of five dogs, and an increased left ventricular systolic and aortic systolic pressure in another dog.[75] Increases of cardiac output, left ventricular stroke volume, and peak blood velocity in the descending aorta were reported in goats at nine months postoperatively.[81,82] Using conditioned latissimus dorsi for ventricular wall replacement in goats, this same group showed no difference in cardiac output between controls and right or left ventricle replacement after six months.[83] In a similar model using dogs, Soberman showed improved right ventricular contractility and ejection fraction during muscle stimulation.[84]

Anderson wrapped normal canine hearts with unconditioned latissimus dorsi grafts.[85] After a 3-week vascular delay, and four months of electrical stimulation, the muscle grafts were able to generate tension as measured by strain gauge, however, with synchronous contraction of the grafts, there was no increase in cardiac output. Three dogs were placed on cardiopulmonary bypass, cardiac fibrillation was induced, and an average increase of only 15 mmHg of left ventricular pressure was noted during muscle contraction.

While the above studies used normal hearts, various cardiac failure models have been studied. Takemura used an onlay graft to support an infarcted right ventricular free wall caused by ligation of the coronary vessels supplying it.[86] Improvements of right ventricular pressure and pulmonary artery pressure were shown with muscle stimulation. A global heart failure model using propranolol has been evaluated by Chagas.[3] After 6-8 weeks of muscle conditioning in a canine, cardiomyoplasty was performed, and heart failure was induced. In this acute setting, with synchronous muscle stimulation, increases of cardiac output, stroke volume, stroke work and ejection fraction were recorded.

An acute model of dilated cardiomyopathy in dogs, induced by rapid ventricular pacing, has also been used to study cardiomyoplasty with unconditioned muscle.[87] Left ventricular wall stress was then calculated using major and minor axis dimensions.[88] Increases of cardiac output and stroke work occurred with muscle stimulation, and wall stress decreased. This suggested that systolic augmentation with cardiomyoplasty was achieved by dynamically altering the left ventricular dimensions, resulting in improved work efficiency.

Determination of the exact mechanism of action of cardiomyoplasty in a heart failure model has been limited due to the unavailability of a chronic heart failure model. Both the propranolol and rapid ventricular pacing models are reversible acute models. Doxorubicin has been used for a chronic failure model but the resultant cardiomyopathy is frequently progressive.[89] Doxorubicin can also produce a fatal gastrointestinal toxicity in the canine.[90] Recently, a sheep model of left ventricular infarction, with reproducible impairment of cardiac function, has been reported[91] Using this model in our laboratory resulted in ventricular aneurysms of 20% heart surface. After cardiomyoplasty with the left latissimus dorsi, contractility, as determined by maximal elastance (E_{max}), improved with the muscle wrap, however, stimulation produced only mild increases of E_{max}.

Because of the lack of a precise understanding of the mechanism of action of cardiomyoplasty, there has been an array of muscle conditioning protocols, electrical stimulation modes and different surgical techniques. The significance of these parameters to the muscle transformation and its subsequent functional performance, have not been defined. However, this non-uniformity makes it difficult to draw conclusions regarding the best method of conditioning. Experimental studies have demonstrated better cardiac augmentation with pulse train stimulation of the muscle graft.[3,36,45,60,81,83,92]

The best technique for wrapping the latissimus dorsi around the heart is also controversial. Magoverns group has compared two different orientations of the left latissimus dorsi in a propranolol induced acute canine heart failure model.[92] Better hemodynamic improvement was obtained when the muscle was wrapped in a circumferential direction around the heart, starting anterior to posterior with the muscle fibers perpendicular to the ventricular septum, compared to wrapping the muscle posterior to anterior with muscle fibers perpendicular to the septum on the dorsal surface and parallel to the septum on the ventral heart surface.

Clinically, the first cardiomyoplasty using muscle stimulation was performed in 1985 by Carpentier.[10] A fibroma was resected from the right and left ventricles of a 37 year old female and replaced with a pedicle graft of latissimus dorsi. Studies with a ^{99m}Tc heart scan on the 30th postoperative day showed an increased ejection fraction from 56% to 69% with muscle stimulation. This improvement in ejection fraction is difficult to explain from our current knowledge of the mechanism of skeletal muscle stimulation since a DDD type cardiac pacemaker was used which delivered only a single electrical impulse to the muscle graft.

In the same year, Magovern resected a ventricular aneurysm in a 45 year old female, and covered the defect with electrically stimulated latissimus dorsi.[93] Six weeks later, Doppler and thallium studies demonstrated a 10% increase of ejection fraction with synchronous pacing. Like Carpentiers patient, only a single electrical impulse was delivered to the muscle graft.

The current clinical indications for cardiomyoplasty are conditions of irreversible and extensive loss of myocardial contractility, such as ischemic or dilated cardiomyopathy, Chagas myocarditis, or myocardial tumors. Although subjective improvement has been noted in most hospital survivors, fewer patients have had measurable improvements in cardiac output or ejection fraction with the stimulator turned on versus off.[1,12,13,85,94]

Carpentiers' group reported an increase of ejection fraction in 2 of 5 patients at 18 to 33 months postoperatively, although all claimed an improved NYHA functional class.[94] They compared reinforcement cardiomyoplasty (muscle wrapped around the heart), to substitution cardiomyoplasty, where the muscle is used to replace ventricular defects created after resection of an aneurysm or tumor.[95] Patients who underwent reinforcement cardiomyoplasty had a mean preoperative ejection fraction of 15.5%, a postoperative ejection fraction of 13.3% without stimulation, and 21.8% with stimulation. In the substitution group, the mean ejection fraction was 18.6% preoperatively and postoperatively, 20.9% and 26.7% without and with stimulation, respectively. All 12 patients remained in NYHA functional class I or II with a mean follow-up period of 18 months.

Delahaye, et al, reported on eleven patients, mostly with end-stage ischemic heart disease, who had cardiomyoplasty.[96] Six of seven patients who were evaluated six months postoperatively had improved functional status and exercise tolerance with stress testing. Measurements of cardiac function and maximal oxygen consumption, however, showed no improvement with muscle stimulation.

Magovern's group has reported their results on five patients.[12,97,98] One patient died of a ventricular arrhythmia. The other four improved symptomatically and three had improved ejection fractions with muscle stimulation.

In contrast to Magoverns' patients with aneurysms, Jatene in Brazil, has used cardiomyoplasty for the treatment of idiopathic dilated cardiomyopathy (11) and Chagas' disease (2).[8,9,99] Significant improvements of left ventricular stroke volume and stroke work index were reported. Jatene showed that the greatest improvements in ejection fraction were seen in patients who had the smallest left ventricular end diastolic volume preoperatively. This is consistent with Laplace's law, in which the ability of skeletal muscle to develop pressure within the spherically shaped heart, is inversely proportional to the radius of curvature. The smaller cardiac diameter and the increased ventricular wall thickness from the muscle wrap result in a lower calculated wall stress.[88,100]

Jatene also compared patients who had cardiomyoplasty to a similar group of sixteen patients who refused cardiomyoplasty. A significant survival advantage was seen in the operated group at 12 months (80.7% versus 42%) and at 18 months (80.7% versus 31.5%).[99]

Krakovsky, of the Soviet Union, has recently reported the results of 19 patients who underwent cardiomyoplasty.[15] Sixteen had ischemic heart disease and were in either functional class III (5) or IV (11). Three others had dilated cardiomyopathy, all were functional class IV. The operative mortality was 16%. At follow-up of 4 months to 3.5 years, there were two additional deaths. All other patients were in functional class I or II. The average ejection fraction in these 14 survivors increased from 29.5% preoperatively, to 39.4% postoperatively. While most clinical reports used a 1:1 or 1:2 muscle:heart stimulation ratio, Krakovsky claims to obtain best results using 1:4 or 1:6 ratios.

The mechanism of cardiac augmentation with cardiomyoplasty is still speculative. It has been suggested that the external wrap of skeletal muscle provides an accessory contractile layer which assists in the ejection of blood.[3,101] This may be supported by recent information comparing right anterior latissimus dorsi cardiomyoplasty to left anterior latissimus cardiomyoplasty.[102] This partially transfers the cardiac workload to the latissimus dorsi, without an increase of myocardial oxygen consumption. Subsequently, this may slow the progression of the underlying cardiomyopathy or even allow some recovery of cardiac function.[103,104]

Although cardiomyoplasty probably does augment systolic ventricular function in some patients, this active process has not been so evident in the majority of patients. As described in our sheep model, E_{max} was increased with muscle wrapping, but during electrical stimulation of the muscle only slight improvement of systolic blood pressure and peak blood flow occurred in one of five sheep. This is compatible with work by Lee,[87,105] and Salmons[106] who suggest that the muscle wrap plays a passive role in altering the loading conditions of the left ventricle with subsequent reduction of wall stress, which improves the myocardial oxygen supply/demand relationship. During diastole, with ventricular filling and dilation, the cardiomyoplasty must also relax. Normally, skeletal muscle relaxation is dependent in part on antagonist muscle contraction. Guiraudon has suggested that inadequate skeletal muscle relaxation may limit the effects of cardiomyoplasty.[107] The inability of the cardiomyoplasty to relax sufficiently to allow optimal diastolic filling may explain why Krakovsky has obtained better results in some patients at lower heart:muscle contraction ratios.

SKELETAL MUSCLE VENTRICLES

The construction of pumping chambers or "ventricles" is the other, and possibly more important, application of skeletal muscles for cardiac assistance (Figure 2). These SMVs have been connected to the systemic and pulmonary circulation of experimental animals and have shown effective cardiac assist when used in synchrony with the heart. Skeletal muscle can be used as a diastolic counterpulsator, by either wrapping the muscle directly around the aorta, developing a pneumatic or hydraulic drive system, or directing blood flow through a SMV connected to the circulation.

Mannion compared the effects of vascular delay and electrical conditioning of SMVs constructed from latissimus dorsi. He tested them contracting against an external hydraulic test circuit.[48] Using a preload of 24 mmhg and an afterload of 80 mmhg, initial pressures of about 200 mmhg, and flows between 400 and 1000 ml/min were obtained. In SMVs constructed without vascular delay or conditioning, flow diminished to zero in minutes. With vascular delay, flow was sustained slightly longer. The SMVs that had first undergone a vascular delay and then conditioning maintained a pressure of 155 mmHg and a flow of 200 ml/min for the entire four hour test period. Mannion then used conditioned SMVs in the systemic circulation as aortic diastolic counterpulsators.[108] During acute experiments stroke work intermediate between the left and right ventricle was generated over 8 hours.

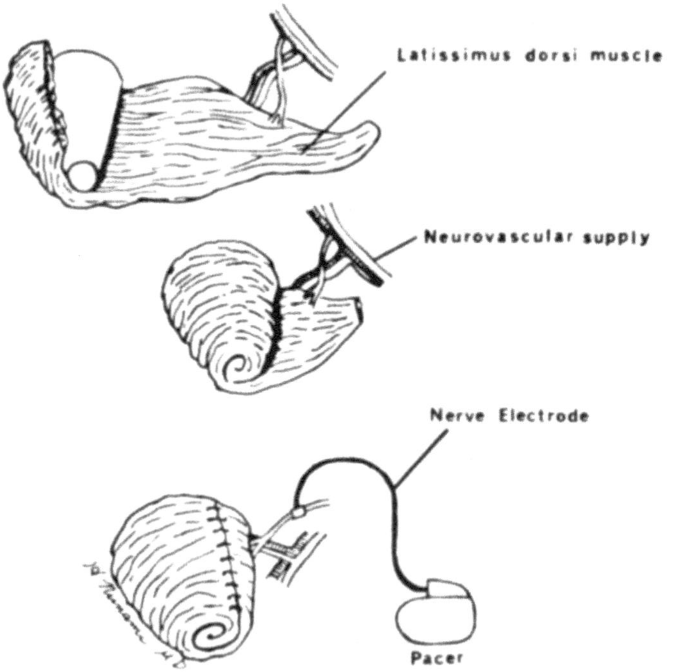

Figure 2. Construction of a skeletal muscle ventricle.

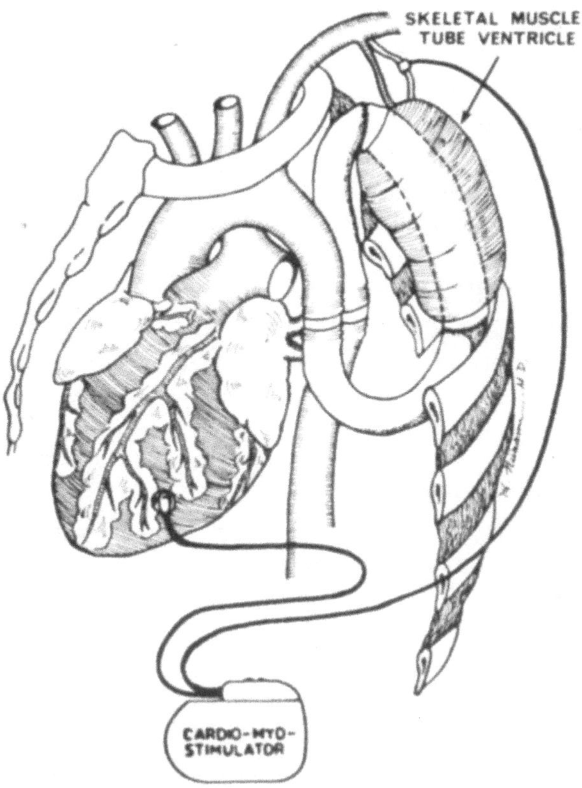

Figure 3. Skeletal muscle tube ventricle at rest.

Following Mannions work, Acker studied the pumping characteristics of a SMV over several weeks using an implantable mock circulation device.[42] Initially, the SMV maintained a systolic pressure of 135 mmHg and a flow of 464 ml/min using a preload of 40 to 50 mmHg and an afterload of 80 mmHg. After 2 weeks of continuous pumping, a pressure of 104 mmHg and a flow of 206 ml/min was generated. However, by varying preload, afterload and burst pattern, these SMVs were capable of systolic pressures of 200 mmHg and flows of 500 ml/min. Two SMVs pumped for five and nine weeks.

In a subsequent experiment, Acker found that electrical preconditioning was not absolutely necessary, at least in the dog, for SMVs to perform sustained work.[44] Six SMVs were constructed, allowed a period of vascular delay, but not electrically conditioned before being called on to perform work. Systolic pressure generated by the SMVs was initially 139 ± 7 mmHg and 107 ± 7 mmHg after one month. Flow was initially 518 ± 105 ml/min and at one month was 224 ± 85 ml/min. Although pressure and flow decreased during one month of continuous pumping, the results indicated that canine skeletal muscle could perform continuous work while simultaneously undergoing adaptive transformation. Furthermore, after two weeks of continuous pumping these SMVs could generate 4.0×10^5 ergs of mean stroke work. Similar work output has been measured in SMVs constructed from the canine rectus abdominis muscle.[79,109]

The effects of electrical preconditioning on skeletal muscle ventricles has been studied by Bridges.[110] Using a mock circulation device, afterloads comparable to the pulmonary and systemic circulation (30 and 80 mmHg) were examined. SMVs preconditioned with continuous 2 Hz stimulation, developed significantly higher stroke work then SMVs conditioned with 25 Hz burst frequency patterns. Passive stretch during preconditioning also contributed to an increased stroke work.[111] With 85 hz burst stimulation, the SMV stroke work averaged 410% of canine right ventricle stroke work and 59% of the canine left ventricle stroke work. Further improvements of stroke work have been achieved using larger volume SMVs.[112] Addition studies have verified that SMVs can generate a stroke work greater than the right ventricle.[42,44,47-49,79,108,113]

In experiments using a SMV as a right heart substitute, Bridges successfully bypassed the right ventricle and maintained a systemic systolic blood pressure of 95 mmHg, after four hours of continuous work.[114]

Acker studied SMVs that pumped blood within the systemic arterial circulation for weeks at a time.[43] The SMV was modified to a flow-though design and connected to the descending thoracic aorta with an interposition graft (Figure 3). Six SMVs were stimulated to contract synchronously during cardiac diastole and functioned chronically as diastolic counterpulsators. The SMV was stimulated via its motor nerve using an implantable prototype R wave synchronous burst stimulator driven by the heart's electrical activity. Awake dogs tolerated these contracting SMVs well and ambulated without apparent difficulty. The animals were tether free in that no tubes or wires crossed the skin. Significant diastolic augmentation was produced by the SMVs for several weeks. The SMVs in this study were not electrically preconditioned. Increase in the slow myosin content of the SMVs from two dogs who survived 5 and 11 weeks showed adaptive transformation of the muscle during continuous pumping. Unfortunately, thromboemboli developed which lead to renal failure and subsequent death.

Anderson constructed SMVs in fifteen dogs. After a delay period of 4 weeks the SMVs were connected to the descending thoracic aorta with a polytetrafluoroethylene bifurcation graft (Figure 4). The aorta was ligated between the two limbs of the graft so that there was obligatory blood flow through the SMV. Nine skeletal muscle ventricles were lined with autogenously derived tissue, either pleura or pericardium, whereas six had no specific lining other than an induced fibrous reaction. The SMVs were activated to contract during cardiac diastole. Aortic diastolic counterpulsation was achieved in all dogs, with ten surviving from 1 week to beyond 9 months. Thrombus eventually developed in all but three of the SMVs, but no dog had clinical evidence of thromboemboli. The three thrombus-free SMVs were lined with pleura, including the animal surviving beyond 9 months. These

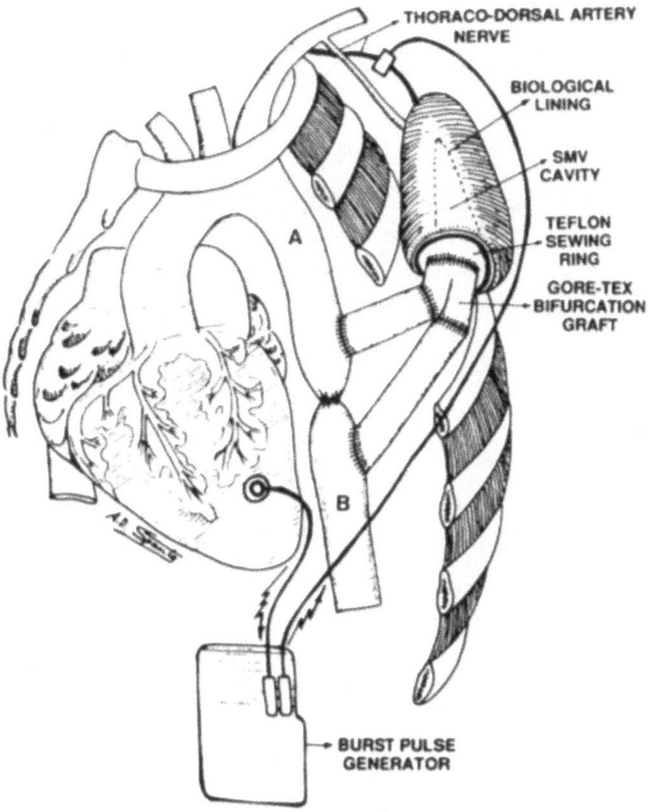

Figure 4. Diagram of skeletal muscle ventricle (SMV) in circulation. The SMV is on the outside of the chest wall. The limbs of the bifurcation graft have been divided to prevent kinking.

results indicated that canine skeletal muscle could provide aortic diastolic counterpulsation for 9 months without clinically apparent thromboembolic complications. An SMV with this configuration remained stable in one animal until a terminal study at 836 days[16,115-117](Figure 5).

Additional modifications have included placement of a valve in the efferent limb of the SMV, which resulted in a marked reduction in left ventricular stroke work associated with augmented coronary blood flow.[118] The effect of timing with an afferent limb valve opening on pre-contraction pressures within a SMV has been studied as a means to understand muscle fatigue.[119] Geddes has found that by restricting blood flow to the SMV, the pre-contraction pressure within the SMV is reduced, and therefore muscle capillary blood flow increases, potentially reducing long-term muscle fatigue. This illustrates the trade off between the need for relatively high filling pressures to optimize SMV stroke work, and the importance of capillary blood flow during SMV relaxation.

Chachques wrapped latissimus dorsi muscle around the ascending aorta and proximal transverse arch in goats[120] The muscle grafts were

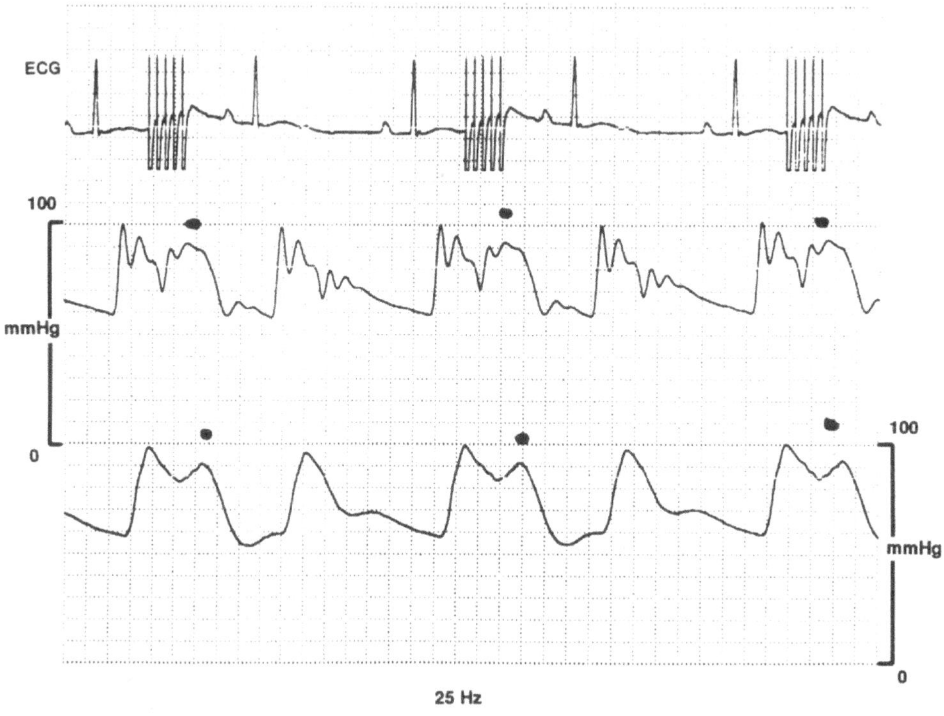

Figure 5. Pressure tracing of skeletal muscle ventricle (SMV) which has been pumping in the circulation for eighteen months with 25 Hz stimulation. Diastolic pressure peak during SMV contraction is marked.

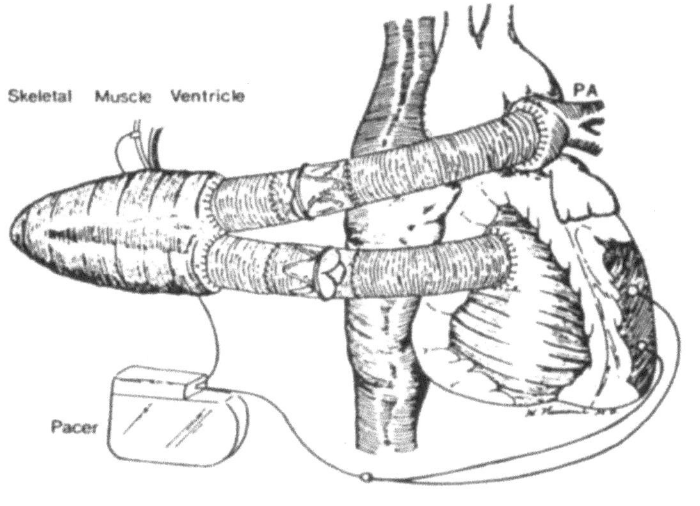

Figure 6. Diagram of skeletal muscle ventricle connected between the right ventricle and pulmonary artery (modified Rastelli configuration).

stimulated during diastole and heart failure was induced with propranolol. The ascending aorta was enlarged in some goats with a glutaraldehyde treated patch of pericardium. Chachques found an increase of the subendocardial viability index,[121] although fatigue occurred within minutes in these unconditioned muscle. Aortic enlargement resulted in a greater percent increase of this index than in animals without aortic enlargement. In acute pilot experiments in our laboratory similar changes have been recorded.

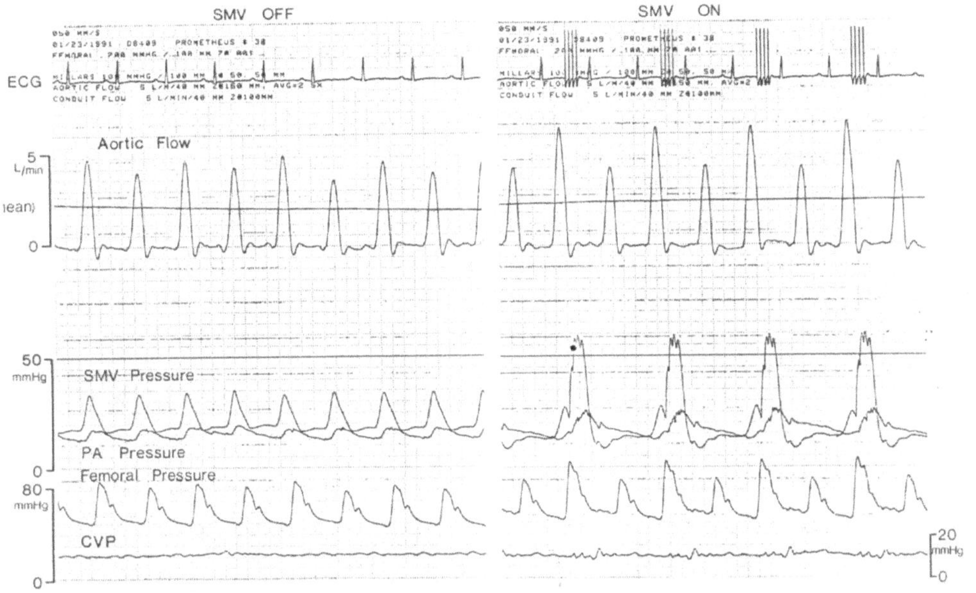

Figure 7. Representative hemodynamic tracings of skeletal muscle ventricle in modified Rastelli configuration.

Other configurations have included using the SMV with valved conduits between the right ventricle and the pulmonary artery (Figure 6,7), and the left atrium and aorta.[122,123] Effective augmentation of pulmonary blood flow has been achieved in the former model for over two months.

Connecting a SMV from the left ventricular apex to the aorta seems to be a particularly promising configuration. In a canine model, with an abdominis rectus SMV, and ß-block induced heart failure, cardiac output increased an average 31% after 30 minutes of assist.[124] In this same configuration, using normal hearts and conditioned latissimus dorsi SMVs, our lab found significant increases of the endocardial viability ratio, systemic blood pressure, and diastolic augmentation. SMV flow was about half of the cardiac output initially, and maintained 85% of this flow after 3 hours in circulation.

Voytik used electronics to model the human circulation as resistive-capacitive networks, with pressures as voltages, blood flow as electrical current, cardiac valves as diodes, heart chambers and great vessels as capacitors, and capillary beds as resistors.[2] This modeling, with simulation of congestive heart failure, has demonstrated the superiority of the left ventricular apico-aortic configuration compared to an aorta-aortic and atrial-aortic design. This also appears to be the preferred configuration used clinically with some mechanical assist devices.[6]

SUMMARY

Research using skeletal muscle for cardiac augmentation has made significant advances in the last two decades primarily due to better understanding of the plasticity of skeletal muscle and because of advances in pacemaker technology. Cardiomyoplasty is now being evaluated as one form of skeletal muscle cardiac assist in patients with heart failure. Symptomatically, the patients have improved, although there has not been consistent improvement of measured hemodynamic parameters. Research continues as to the actual mechanism of cardiac assistance with cardiomyoplasty.

The potential for human use of skeletal muscle ventricles appears promising, particularly with the success in a long term animal model beyond two years. Several issues must by resolved however. It is not known whether muscle fibrosis, found in some earlier studies, is progressive or not. However, in muscles in situ stimulated continuously for 1 year, no muscle damage was observed.[63,125] Finally, the optimal configuration for SMVs in the circulation needs further study, and problems of blood-nonendothelial cell surface interaction, flow direction, and requirements for valved conduits must be addressed.

ACKNOWLEDGEMENTS

Supported by the National Institute of Health Grant HL 34778.

REFERENCES

1. A.B. Hill, R.C.-J. Chiu. Dynamic cardiomyoplasty for treatment of heart failure. *Clin Cardiol* 12:681-688;1989.
2. S.L. Voytik, C.F. Babbs, S.F. Badylak. Simple electrical model of the circulation of explore design parameters for a skeletal muscle ventricle. *J Heart Trans* 9:160-174;1990.
3. A.C.P. Chagas, L.F.P. Moreira, G.P. Camarano, P.L. da Luz, A. Leirner, N.A.G. Stolf, A.D. Jatene. Stimulated preconditioned skeletal muscle cardiomyoplasty: an effective means of cardiac assist. *Circulation* 80:III-202-208;1989.

4. W.J. Kolff. The artificial heart, the inevitable development: will it be the U.S., or abroad? *Artif Organs* 13:183-184;1989.
5. J.A. Franciosa, M. Wilen, S. Zieseke, et al: Survival in men with severe chronic left ventricular failure due to either coronary artery or idiopathic dilated cardiomyopathy. *Am J of Cardio* 51:831;1983.
6. P.M. McCarthy, P.M. Portner, H.G. Toble, V.A. Starnes, N. Ramasamy, P.E. Oyer. Clinical experience with the Novacor ventricular assist system. *J Thorac Cardiovasc Surg* 102:578-587;1991.
7. L. Molteni, H.E. Almada, C. de Palma and R. Ferreira. Dynamic cardiomyoplasty: Clinical experience. In: *Transformed Muscle for Cardiac Assist and Repair*, Edited by R.C-Y Chiu, Bourgeois, I.M., Mount Kisco, Futura Publishing Co.Inc.;1989.
8. A.D. Jatene, L.F.P. Moreira, N.A.G. Stolf, E.A. Bocchi, P. Seferian,Jr., P.M.P. Fernandes, H. Abensur: Left ventricular function changes after cardiomyoplasty in patients with dilated cardiomyopathy. *J Thorac Cardiovasc Surg* 102:132-139;1991.
9. L.F.P. Moreira and A.D. Jatene. Cardiomyoplasty in dilated cardiomyopathy. In: *Cardiomyoplasty* edited by Carpentier, A., Chachques, J.C. and Grandjean, P., Mount Kisco, Futura Publishing Co.Inc., p. 171-179:1991.
10. A. Carpentier, J.C. Chachques. Myocardial substitution with a stimulated skeletal muscle: first successful clinical case. *Lancet* 1:1267;1985.
11. J.C. Chachques, P.A. Grandjean, A. Carpentier. Patient management and clinical follow-up after cardiomyoplasty. *J Card Surg* 6:89-99;1991.
12. G.J. Magovern, S.B. Park, R.L. Kao, I.Y. Christlieb, G.J. Magovern, Jr: Dynamic cardiomyoplasty in patients. *J Heart Trans* 9:258-263;1990.
13. G.J. Magovern, I.Y. Christlieb, R.L. Kao. The Allegheny hospital experience. In: *Cardiomyoplasty* edited by A. Carpentier, J.C. Chachques, and P. Grandjean, Mount Kisco, Futura Publishing Co.Inc, p.159-170;1991.
14. A.S. Dumcius, E.K. Sirvinskas, J. Skucas, K.M. Salcius, A.A. Krakovsky, S.J. Giedraitis, V.S. Chekanov. A method of extended myoventriculoplasty with programmable cardiosynchronized electroneurostimulation: description and initial clinical results. *Cora Vasa* 31(5):394-401;1989.
15. A.A. Krakovsky, V.V. Pekarsky, A.S. Dumcius, V.I. Merzlijakov, D.B. Andreev, A.M. Dijadurko, V.V. Piluiko, L.G. Rijabinia, R. Fietsam,Jr., I.A. Dubrovsky, A.N. Rijich, V.S. Chekanov. Latissimus dorsi cardiomyoplasty: the Russian experimental and clinical data. *J Heart Trans* submitted;1991.
16. F.W. Mocek, D.R. Anderson, A. Pochettino, R.L. Hammond, A.D. Spanta, G.L. Thomas, H. Lu, R. Fietsam,Jr., H Nakajima, A. Krakovsky, T.L. Hooper, H. Niinami, M. Colson, S. Levine, L.W. Stephenson. Skeletal Muscle Ventricles in Circulation Long-Term: 191 to 836 Days. *J Heart Transplant* 1991.(In Press)
17. F.R. de Jesus. Breve consideraciones sobre un case de herida penetrante del corazon. *Bol Assoc Med Puerto Rcio* 23:380-382;1931.
18. R. Leriche. Essai experimental de traitement de certains infarctus du myocarde et de l'aneurisme de coeur par une graffe muscle strie. *Bull Soc Nat Chir* 9:229-232;1933.
19. C.S. Beck. A new blood supply to the heart by operation. *Surg Gynecol Obstet* 61:407-410;1935.
20. C.S. Beck. The development of a new blood supply to the heart by operation. *Ann Surg* 102:801-810;1935.
21. L. O'Shaughnessy. Experimental method of providing a collateral circulation to the heart. *Brit J Surg* 23:665;1936.
22. C.S. Beck. Further data on the establishment of a new blood supply to the heart by operation. *J Thorac Surg* 5:604-611;1936.

23. C.S. Beck. Coronary sclerosis and angina pectoris: Treatment by grafting a new blood supply upon the myocardium. *Surg Gynecol Obstet* 64:270-272; 1937.
24. B.V. Petrovsky. The use of diaphragmatic flaps for plastic purpose in thoracic surgery. *Chest Surgery (Moscow)* 51:73-80;1959.
25. B.V. Petrovsky. Certain problems of surgical treatment in cardiac aneurysms. *Surgery (Moscow)* 4:11-39;1959.
26. B.V. Petrovsky. Surgical treatment of cardiac aneurysms following myocardial infarction. *Surgery (Moscow)* 9:11-20;1960.
27. B.V. Petrovsky. The use of the diaphragm graft for plastic operations in thoracic surgery. *J Thorac Cardiovasc Surg* 41:348-355;1961.
28. B.V. Petrovsky. The surgical treatment of cardiac aneurysms. *Surgery (Moscow)* 2:5-14;1963.
29. B.V. Petrovsky. Surgical treatment of cardiac aneurysms. *J Cardiovasc Surg* 2:87-91;1966.
30. M.D. Papp. Experimental use of intercostal muscle flaps for repair of induced cardiac defects. *J Thorac Cardiovasc Surg* 90:261;1985.
31. H.V. Schaff, P.G. Arnold, G.S. Reeder. Late mediastinal infection and pseudoaneurysm following left ventricular aneurysmectomy repair utilizing pectoralis major muscle flap. *J Thorac Cardiovasc Surg* 84:912-916;1982.
32. A. Kantrowitz, W. McKinnon. The experimental use of the diaphragm as an auxiliary myocardium. *Surg Forum* 9:266-268;1959.
33. A. Kantrowitz. Functioning autogenous muscle used experimentally as an auxiliary ventricle. *Trans Am Soc Artif Intern Organs* 68:305-307;1960.
34. E. Kusaba, W. Schraut, S. Sawatani. A diaphragmatic graft for augmenting left ventricular function: a feasibility study. *Trans Am Soc Artif Intern Organs* 19:251-257;1973.
35. K. Nakamura, W.W.L. Glenn. Graft of the diaphragm as a functioning substitute for the myocardium. *J Surg Res* 4:435-439;1964.
36. M.L. Dewar, D.C. Drinkwater, C. Wittnich, R.C.-J. Chiu. Synchronously stimulated skeletal muscle graft for myocardial repair. *J Thorac Cardiovasc Surg* 87:325-331;1984.
37. H. Termet, J.L. Chalencon, E. Estour, et al. Transplantation sur le myocarde d'un muscle strie excité pace maker. *Ann Chir Thorac Cardiovasc* 5:568;1966.
38. W.I. Hume. Construction of a functioning accessory myocardium. *Trans Southern Surg Assoc* 79:200-202;1968.
39. H.M. Spotnitz, C. Merker, J.R. Malm. Applied physiology of the canine rectus abdominis: Force-length curves correlated with functional characteristics of a rectus powered "ventricle": Potential for cardiac assistance. *Trans Am Soc Artif Intern Organs* 20:747-756;1974.
40. A. von Recum, J.P. Stule, O. Hamada, et al: Long-term stimulation of diaphragm muscle pouch. *J Surg Res* 23:422-427;1977.
41. F.R. Adams and A. Schwartz. Comparative mechanisms for contraction of cardiac and skeletal muscle. *Chest* 78:123-139;1980.
42. M.A. Acker, R.L. Hammond, J.D. Mannion, S. Salmons, L.W. Stephenson. An Autologous Biologic Pump Motor. *J Thorac Cardiovasc Surg* 94:733-746; 1986.
43. M.A. Acker, W.A. Anderson, R.L. Hammond, A.J. Chin, J.W. Buchanan, C.C. Morse, A.M. Kelly, L.W. Stephenson. Skeletal muscle ventricles in circulation: one to eleven weeks' experience. *J Thorac Cardiovasc Surg* 94:163-174;1987.
44. M.A. Acker, R.L. Hammond, J.D. Mannion, S. Salmons, L.W. Stephenson. Skeletal muscle as the potential power source for a cardiovascular pump: assessment in vivo. *Science* 236:324-327;1987.

45. M.L. Dewar, R.C.-J. Chiu. Cardiomyoplasty and the pulse-train stimulator. In: *Biomechanical Cardiac Assist: Cardiomyoplasty and Muscle-powered Devices*, edited by R.C-J Chiu, New York: Futura, p. 43-58;1986.
46. D.C. Drinkwater, R.C.-J. Chiu, D. Modry, et al: Cardiac assist and myocardial repair with synchronously stimulated skeletal muscle. *Surg Forum* 31:271-273;1980.
47. J.D. Mannion, R.L. Hammond, M.A. Acker, L.W. Stephenson. Four hour circulatory assistance with canine skeletal muscle ventricles. *Surg Forum* 37:211-213;1986.
48. J. Mannion, R.L. Hammond, L.W. Stephenson. Hydraulic pouches of canine latissimus dorsi: Potential for left ventricular assistance. *J Thorac Cardiovasc Surg* 91:534-544;1986.
49. B.R. Vachon, J. Kunov, W. Zingg: Mechanical properties of diaphragm muscle in dogs. *Med Biol Eng* 13:252-260;1975.
50. J.C. Buller, J.C. Eccles, R.M. Eccles. Differentiation of fast and slow muscles in the cat hind limb. *J Physiol* 150:399-416;1960.
51. J.C. Buller, J.C. Eccles, R.M. Eccles. Interactions between motor neurons and muscles in respect of the characteristic speeds of their responses. *J Physiol* 150:417-439;1960.
52. S. Salmons, G. Vrbova. The influence of activity on some contractile characteristics of mammalian fast and slow muscles. *J Physiol* 210:535-549;1969.
53. S. Salmons, F.A. Sreter. Significance of impulse activity in the transformation of skeletal muscle type. *Nature* 263:30-34;1976.
54. M.M.Y. Chi, C.S. Hintz, J. Henriksson, et al. Chronic stimulation of mammalian muscle: Enzyme changes in individual fibers. *J Physiol* 251:C633-C642;1986.
55. D. Pette. Activity-induced fast to slow transitions in mammalian muscle. *Med Sci Sports Exerc* 16:517-528;1984.
56. S. Salmons, J. Henriksson. The adaptive response of skeletal muscle to increased use. *Muscle Nerve* 4:94;1981.
57. P. Schantz, R. Billeter, J. Henriksson, E. Jansson. Training-induced increase in myofibrillar ATPase intermediate fibers in human skeletal muscle. *Muscle Nerve* October:628-636;1982.
58. B.R. Eisenberg, S. Salmons. The reorganization of subcellular structure in muscle undergoing fast-to-slow type transformation. *Cell Tissue Res* 220:449;1981.
59. D. Pette, W. Muller, E. Leisner, G. Vrbova. Time dependent effects on contractile properties, fibre population, myosin light change and enzymes of energy metabolism in intermittently and continuously stimulated fast twitch muscle of the rabbit. *Pfluegers Arch* 364:103;1976.
60. L.C. Permut, I.L. Siegman, J.A. Swain, R.E. Clark. Hemodynamic effects of chronically stimulated skeletal muscle on the dysfunctional canine left ventricle. *Surg Forum* 39:278-280;1988.
61. C.D. Ianuzzo, N. Hamilton, P.J. O'Brien, T. Dionisopoulos, T. Salerno, R.C.-J. Chiu. Biochemical character of cardiac and transformed canine skeletal muscle. In: *Transformed Muscle for Cardiac Assist and Repair*, edited by R.C-Y Chiu and Bourgeois, I.M. Mount Kisco, Futura Publishing Co.Inc.;1989.
62. O. Hudlicka, M. Brown, M. Cotter, M. Smith, G. Vrbova. The effect of long-term stimulation of fast muscle on their blood flow. *Pfluegers Arch* 369:141-149;1977.
63. C.N. Mayne, W.A. Anderson, R.L. Hammond, B.R. Eisenberg, L.W. Stephenson, S. Salmons. Correlates of fatigue resistance in canine skeletal muscle stimulated electrically for up to one year. *Am J Physiol* 261(2 Pt 1):C259-C270;1991.

64. R.C.-J. Chiu, G. Kochamba, G. Walsh, M. Dewar, C. Dewrosiers, T. Dionisopoulos, P. Brady, C.D. Ianuzzo. Biochemical and functional correlates of myocardium-like transformed skeletal muscle as a power source for cardiac assist devices. *J Card Surg* 4(2):171;1989.
65. M.J. Dawson, D.G. Gadian, D.R. Wilkie. Mechanical relaxation rate and metabolism studied in fatiguing muscle by phosphorus nuclear magnetic resonance. *J Physiol Lond* 299:465-484;1980.
66. E. Leberer, U. Seedorf, D. Pette. Neural control of gene expression in skeletal muscle. Calcium-sequestering proteins in developing and chronically stimulated rabbit skeletal muscles. *Biochem J* 239:295-300; 1986.
67. M.A. Acker, W.A. Anderson, R.L. Hammond et al. Oxygen consumption of fatigue-resistant muscle. *J Thorac Cardiovasc Surg* 94:702-709;1987.
68. B.J. Clark, M.A. Acker, K. McCully, H. Subramanian, R.L. Hammond, S. Salmons, B. Chance, L.W. Stephenson. In vivo P-NMR spectroscopy of chronically stimulated canine skeletal muscle. *Am J Physiol* 254:C258-C266; 1988.
69. F.R. Armenti, T. Bitto, J.A. Macoviak, A.M. Kelly, C.T. Chase, B.K. Hoffman, N.A. Rubenstein, M. St.John-Sutton, L.H. Edmunds,Jr., L.W. Stephenson. Transformation of Canine Diaphragm to fatigue-Resistant Muscle by Phrenic Nerve Stimulation. *Surg Forum* 35:258-269;1984.
70. J.A. Macoviak, L.W. Stephenson, A. Alavi, A.M. Kelly, L.H. Edmunds,Jr. Effect of Electrical Stimulation on Diaphragmatic Muscle used to Enlarge Right Ventricle. *Surgery* 90:271-277;1981.
71. J.A. Macoviak, L.W. Stephenson, F. Armenti, A.M. Kelly, A. Alavi, T. Mackler, J. Cox, G.M. Palatianos, L.H. Edmunds,Jr., Electrical Conditioning of *in situ* Skeletal Muscle for Replacement of Myocardium. *J Surg Res.* 32:429-439;1982.
72. J.D. Mannion, T. Bitto, R.L. Hammond, N. Rubinstein, L.W. Stephenson. Histochemical and Fatigue Characteristics of Conditioned Latissimus Dorsi Muscle. *Circ Res* 58:298-30;1986.
73. E. Hohenhaus, W.A. Anderson, A. Pochettino, D.R. Anderson, H. Niinami, A.D. Spanta, R.L. Hammond, C.R. Bridges,Jr., L.W. Stephenson. Skeletal Muscle for Cardiac Assistance. In: *Cardiac Surgery: State of the Art Reviews* Vol 4, No 3, Hanley & Belfus, Inc. p 677-702;1990.
74. B.K. Hoffman, B. Gambke, L.W. Stephenson, N.A. Rubenstein. Myosin transitions in chronic stimulation do not involve embryonic isozymes. *Muscle Nerve* 8:796-805;1985.
75. J.C. Chachques, V. Mitz, M. Hero, P. Arhan, P. Galliz, F. Fontrliran, R. Vilain. Experimental cardioplasty using the Latissimus Dorsi muscle flap. *J Cardiovasc Surg* 26:457-462;1985.
76. J.E. Christ, M. Spira. Application of the latissimus dorsi muscle to the heart. *Ann Plast Surg* 8:118-121;1982.
77. J.K.G. Laitung, F. Peck. Shoulder function following loss of the latissimus dorsi muscle. *Br J Plastic Surg* 38:375-379;1985.
78. S. Salmons, J.C. Jarvis. The working capacity of skeletal muscle transformed for use in a cardiac assist role. In: *Transformed skeletal muscle for cardiac assist and repair*, edited by R.C-Y Chiu, I.M. Bourgeois, Mount Kisco, NY: Futura Publishing Company Inc., p. 89-104;1990.
79. J.D. Mannion, M. Velchick, M.A. Acker, R.L. Hammond, A. Alavi, L.W. Stephenson. Transmural Blood Flow to Multi-layered Latissimus Dorsi Skeletal Muscle Ventricles During Circulatory Assistance. *Trans.Amer.Soc.Artif.Intern.Organs* 32:454-460;1986.
80. J.D. Mannion, M. Velchick, R.L. Hammond et al. Effects of collateral blood vessel ligation and electrical conditioning on blood flow in dog latissimus dorsi. *J Surg Res* 47:332-340;1989.

81. J.C. Chachques, P.A. Grandjean, K. Schwartz, S. Mihaileanu, M. Fardeau, B. Swynghedauw, F. Fontaliran, N. Romero, C. Wisnewsky, P. Perier, S. Chauvaud, I.M. Bourgeois, A. Carpentier. Effect of latissimus dorsi dynamic cardiomyoplasty on ventricular function. *Circulation* 78(Suppl III):III-203-III-216;1988.
82. J.C. Chachques, P.A. Grandjean, P. Nataf, S. Mihaileanu, P. Perier, I.M. Bourgeois, A. Carpentier. Dynamic cardiomyoplasty: a surgical approach for ventricular assistance. *Int J Artif Organ* 11:469-474;1988.
83. J.C. Chachques, P.A. Grandjean, J.J. Tommasi, P. Perier, S. Chauvaud, I.M. Bourgeois, A. Carpentier. Dynamic Cardiomyoplasty: A new approach to assist chronic myocardial failure. *Life Support Systems* 5:323-327;1987.
84. M.S. Soberman, I.L Wornom,III., A.G. Justicz, J.J. Coleman,III, G.E. Austin, N.P. Alazraki and J.D. Sink. Latissimus dorsi dynamic cardiomyoplasty of the right ventricle. *J Thorac Cardiovasc Surg* 99:817-827;1990.
85. W.A. Anderson, J.S. Andersen, M.A. Acker, R.L. Hammond, A.J. Chin, P.S. Douglas, A. Khalafalla, S. Salmons and L.W. Stephenson. Skeletal Muscle Applied to the Heart: A Word of Caution. *Circulation* 78 (III):180-190; 1988.
86. H. Takemura, G. Watanabe, N. Sakakibara et al. Ventricular assistance by right free wall dynamic cardiomyoplasty following acute right heart failure in canines. *J Card Surg* 6:132;1991.
87. K.F. Lee, R.J. Dignan, J.M. Parmar, C.M. Dyke, G. Brenton, J Yeh,Jr., A.S. Abd-Elfattah, A.S. Wechsler. Effects of dynamic cardiomyoplasty of left ventricular performance and myocardial mechanics in dilated cardiomyopathy. *J Thorac Cardiovasc Surg* 102:124-131;1991.
88. H. Sandler, H.T. Dodge. Left ventricular tension and stress in man. *Circ.Res.* 13:91-104;1963.
89. R. Danesi, M.D. Tacca, N. Bernardini, G. Cardini, O. Bellini. Evaluation of the JT and corrected JT intervals as a new ECG method for monitoring doxorubicin cardiotoxicity in the dog. *J Pharm Methods* 21:317-327;1989.
90. E.H. Herman, V.J. Ferrans, R.S.K. Young, R.L. Hamlin. Effect of pretreatment with ICRF-187 on the total cumulative dose of doxorubicin tolerated by beagle dogs. *Cancer Res* 48:6918-6925;1988.
91. R.W.J. Millner, J.M. Mann, I. Pearson, J.R. Pepper. Experimental model of left ventricular failure. *Ann Thorac Surg* 52:78;1991.
92. R.L. Kao, I.Y. Christlieb, G.J. Magovern, S.B. Park, G.J. Magovern,Jr.: The importance of skeletal muscle fiber orientation for dynamic cardiomyoplasty. *J Thorac Cardiovasc Surg* 99:134-140;1990.
93. G.J. Magovern, S.B. Park, G.J. Magovern,Jr., D.H. Benckart, G. Tullis, E. Rozar, R.L. Kao, I.Y. Christlieb. Latissimus dorsi as a functioning synchronously paced muscle component in the repair of a left ventricular aneurysm. *Ann Thorac Surg* 41:116;1986.
94. A.A. Hagege, M. Desnos, J.C. Chachques et al. Preliminary report: follow-up after dynamic cardiomyoplasty. *Lancet* 335:1122;1990.
95. J.C. Chachques, P.A. Grandjean, T.A. Pfeffer, P. Perier, G. Dreyfus, V. Jebara, C. Acar, M. Levy, I.M. Bourgeois, J-N. Fabiani, A. Deloche, A. Carpentier. Cardiac assistance by atrial or ventricular cardiomyoplasty. *J Heart Trans* 9:239-251;1990.
96. F. Delahaye, O. Jegaden, P. Montagna et al. Latissimus dorsi cardiomyoplasty in severe congestive heart failure: the Lyon experience. *Circulation* 82(Suppl III):713;1990.
97. G.J. Magovern, F.R. Heckler, S.B. Park, I.Y. Christlieb, G.J. Magovern,Jr., R.L. Kao, D.H. Benckart, G. Tullis, E. Rozar, G.A. Liebler, J. Burkholder, T.D. Maher. Paced latissimus dorsi used for dynamic cardiomyoplasty of left ventricular aneurysms. *Ann Thorac Surg* 44:379-388;1987.
98. G.J. Magovern, F.R. Heckler, S.B. Park, I.Y. Christlieb, G.A. Liebler, J.A. Burkholder, T.D. Maher, D.H. Benckart, G.J. Magovern,Jr., R.L. Kao.

Paced skeletal muscle for dynamic cardiomyoplasty. *Ann Thorac Surg* 45:614-619;1988.

99. L.F.P. Moreira, P. Seferian, E.A. Bocchi, P.M.P. Fernandes, N.A.G. Stolf, A.C.P. Barreto, A.D. Jatene. Survival improvement with dynamic cardiomyoplasty in patients with dilated cardiomyopathy. *Circulation* 82 (Suppl III):713;1990.

100. K.F. Lee, C.M. Dyke, R.J. Dignan, G.S. Benton, A.S. Wechsler. Mechanism of systolic augmentation in dynamic cardiomyoplasty. *Surg Forum* 42:310-3-11;1991.

101. S. Salmons, J.C. Jarvis. Cardiomyoplasty: the basic issues. *Cardiac Chronicle* 4(2):1-6;1990.

102. A.P. Furnary, J.A. Magovern, I.Y. Christlieb, D.R. Trumble. Improved ventricular augmentation with right latissimus dorsi cardiomyoplasty. *Surg Forum* 42:307-309;1991.

103. L. Molteni, H.E. Almada, R.F. Ferreira, D. Ortega. Assessment of the optimal time interval between QRS and single-pulse stimulation in dynamic cardiomyoplasty. In: *Transformed Muscle for Cardiac Assist and Repair*, edited by Chiu, R.C-J. and Bourgeois, I.M. Mount Kisco, Futura, p. 189-196;1990.

104. L.W. Stevenson, J.K. Perloff. The dilated cardiomyopathies: clinical aspects. In: *Cardiology Clinics; vol 2: The cardiomyopathies*, edited by Perloff, J.K. Philadelphia: WB Saunders, p. 187-218;1988.

105. K.F. Lee, C.M. Dyke, A.S. Wechsler. Theoretical considerations in the use of dynamic cardiomyoplasty to treat dilated cardiomyopathy. *J Card Surg* 6:119-123;1991.

106. S. Salmons, J.C. Jarvis. Cardiomyoplasty: a look at the fundamentals. In: Cardiomyoplasty, edited by A. Carpentier, J.C. Chachques, P.A. Grandjean, Mount Kisco, Futura Publishing Co,Inc. p 3-17;1991.

107. G.M. Guiraudon, T. Morell, D.R. Boughner, D.G. McLellan, A.D. Sharma, W.J. Kostuk and C. Guiraudon. Right ventricular free wall dynamic cardiomyoplasty on a canine chronic right ventricular failure model: Primary report. In: *Transformed Muscle for Cardiac Assist and Repair*, edited by R.C-J Chiu, I.M. Bourgeois, Mount Kisco, Futura Publishing Co.Inc.;1989.

108. J.D. Mannion, M.A. Acker, R.L. Hammond, W. Faltemeyer, S. Duckett, L.W. Stephenson. Power Output of Skeletal Muscle Ventricles in Circulation: Short-term studies. *Circulation* 76:155-162;1987.

109. L. Stevens and J. Brown. Can non-cardiac muscle provide useful cardiac assistance? *Am Surg* 52:423-427;1986.

110. C.R. Bridges,Jr., W.E. Brown, R.L. Hammond, D.R. Anderson, W.A. Anderson, F. DiMeo, L.W. Stephenson. Skeletal Muscle Ventricles: Improved Performance at Physiologic Preloads. *Surgery* 106:275-282;1989.

111. C.R. Bridges,Jr., R.L. Hammond, D.R. Anderson, L.W. Stephenson. Skeletal Muscle Ventricle Mechanics: Effects of Passive Stretch. In: Cardiomyoplasty, edited by Carpentier, A., Chachques, P.A. and Grandjean, P.A. Mount Kisco, Futura Publishing Co. Inc. p 217-225;1991.

112. R.L. Hammond, C.R. Bridges,Jr., F. DiMeo, L.W. Stephenson. Performance of Skeletal Muscle Ventricles: Effects of Ventricular Chamber Size. *J Heart Transplant* 9:252-257;1990.

113. W.A. Anderson, J.S. Andersen, C.R. Bridges,Jr., R.L. Hammond, F. DiMeo, E.E. Frisch, S. Salmons, L.W. Stephenson. Skeletal Muscle Ventricles as a Potential Right Heart Assist or Substitute. *Trans Amer Soc Artif Intern Organs* 34:241-246;1988.

114. C.R. Bridges,Jr., R.L. Hammond, F. DiMeo, L.W. Stephenson. Functional Right Heart Replacement with Skeletal Muscle Ventricles. *Circulation* 80 (Suppl III):183-191;1989.

115. D.R. Anderson, A. Pochettino, R.L. Hammond, E. Hohenhaus, A.D. Spanta, C.R. Bridges,Jr., S. Lavine, M. Colson, L.W. Stephenson. Autogenously Lined Skeletal Muscle Ventricles in Circulation: Up to Nine Months Experience. *J Thorac Cardiovasc Surg* 101:661-670;1991.

116. D.R. Anderson, A. Pochettino, R.L. Hammond, E. Hohenhaus, A.D. Spanta, C.R. Bridges,Jr., S. Lavine, M. Colson, L.W. Stephenson. Autogenously Lined Skeletal Muscle Ventricles in Circulation: Up to Nine Months Experience. *J Thorac Cardiovasc Surg* 101:661-670;1991.

117. R. Ruggiero, D.R. Anderson, H. Niinami, A. Pochettino, T.L. Hooper, R.L. Hammond, S. Lavine, A.D. Spanta, H. Lu, L.W. Stephenson. Skeletal Muscle Ventricles in Circulation: 24-month update. *BAM* 1991.(In Press)

118. T.L. Hooper, R.L. Hammond, H. Niinami, H. Lu, H Nakajima, R. Ruggiero, L.W. Stephenson. Aortic Counterpulsation with a Valved Skeletal Muscle Ventricle: Short-term studies of coronary flow and left ventricular function. *J Thorac Cardiovasc Surg* 1991.(In Press)

119. L.A. Geddes, J.L. Wessale, S.F. Badylak, W. Janas, W.A. Tacker, W.D. Voorhees,III: The use of an electrically activated valve to control preload and provide maximal muscle blood flow with a skeletal-muscle ventricle. *Pace* 13:783-795;1990.

120. J.C. Chachques, P.A. Grandjean, E.I.C. Fischer, C. Latremouille, V.A. Jebara, I.M. Bourgeois, A. Carpentier. Dynamic aortomyoplasty to assist left ventricular failure. *Ann Thorac Surg* 49:225-230;1990.

121. I.R. Neilson, S.J. Brister, A.S. Khalafalla, R.C.-J. Chiu. Left ventricular assistance in dogs using a skeletal muscle powered device for diastolic augmentation. *J Heart Trans* 4:343-347;1985.

122. H. Niinami, T.L. Hooper, R.L. Hammond, R. Ruggiero, A. Pochettino, M. Colson and L.W. Stephenson. A New Configuration for Right Ventricular Assist with Skeletal Muscle Ventricle: Short term studies. *Circulation* Vol 84: 2470-2475;1991.(In Press)

123. T.L. Hooper, H. Niinami, R.L. Hammond, H. Lu, R. Ruggiero, A. Pochettino, L.W. Stephenson. Skeletal Muscle Ventricles as Left Atrial–Aortic Pumps: Short-Term Studies. *Ann Thorac Surg* 54: 316-22; 1992.

124. L.Stevens, S.F. Badylak, W. Janas, M.H. Gray, L.A. Geddes, W.D. Voorhees,III: A skeletal muscle ventricle made from rectus abdominis muscle in the dog. *J Surg Res* 46:84-89;1989.

125. M.A. Acker, J.D. Mannion, W.E. Brown, S. Salmons, J. Henriksson, T. Bitto, D.R. Gale, R.L. Hammond and L.W. Stephenson: Canine diaphragm muscle after one year of continuous electrical stimulation: its potential as a myocardial substitute. *J Appl Physiol* 62:1264-1270;1987.

THORACIC TRANSPLANTATION

G. Michael Deeb, M.D., Steven F. Bolling, M.D., Edward L. Bove, M.D., Louis A. Brunsting, M.D., F. Mark Lupinetti, M.D., and Mark B. Orringer, M.D.

Department of Thoracic Surgery
University of Michigan Hospital
Ann Arbor, Michigan

HISTORY

James Hardy performed the first human heart transplant in 1964 by implanting a primate heart into a human recipient.[1] Although the patient did not survive, this demonstrated that a human being could receive a heart transplant and that the heart was capable of electro-mechanical coupling with the ejection of blood. In 1966 Richard Lower performed the "mirror image" operation by implanting a human donor heart into a primate demonstrating the ability of a human heart to be extracted, cold preserved, and re-implanted in a denervated state with complete electro-mechanical function.[2] In 1967 Christian Barnard completed the first human to human heart transplant in Cape Town, South Africa.[3] One hundred and two heart transplants were performed in 17 centers over the next year with poor results.[4] It was quite evident that transplantation was technically feasible but there were significant deficits in the medical knowledge available for patient management.

For the next ten years the majority of heart transplants were performed at Stanford University.[5,6] With the introduction of the endomyocardial biopsy,[7] improved preservation with cardioplegia, and significant developments in immunosuppression such as polyclonal antilymphocytic[8] therapy and Cyclosporine[9] the transplant procedure progressed from a clinical experimental curiosity to a therapeutic endeavor. By the mid 1980's the number of heart transplant centers in the United States escalated from the mid teens to over one hundred.[10]

Heart-lung transplantation was first conceptualized by Alexis Carrel in 1905[11] and the first clinical heart-lung transplantation was performed by Denton Cooley in 1968.[12] However, clinical success was

Cardiac Surgery: Current Issues, Edited by A.C. Cernaianu and A.J. DelRossi Plenum Press, New York, 1992

thwarted by poor preservation, bronchial dehiscence, and poor immunosuppressant therapy. In 1980, Bruce Reitz had the first long term primate survivors using Cyclosporine therapy and one year later he performed the first long term successful human heart-lung procedure.[13] Throughout the 1980's this procedure gained momentum until the end of the decade when single and double lung transplantation became popular.

Lung transplantation was developed in the laboratory in the 1950's by Metras.[14] In 1963, James Hardy performed the first clinical lung transplant and the patient survived 18 days.[15] Dermon performed a single lung transplant in 1968 and the patient survived 10 months.[16] In 1978, Joel Cooper popularized the omental flap technique to the airway anastomoses for neo-vascularization[17,18] and by 1986 he had the first long-term survivors for single lung transplantation.[19] Alex Patterson popularized the en-bloc double lung procedure in 1987 and by 1989, double lung transplantation was converted to a bilateral single lung procedure.[20]

TRANSPLANT IMMUNOLOGY

The transplant immune response is elicited by proteins on the cell surface of transplanted tissues. These surface proteins are called the major histocompatibility antigens (MHC) and are coded on the sixth chromosome. The MHC proteins define tissue antigenicity from one individual to another and serve to regulate the immune response. There are two major classes of MHC antigens. Class-1 antigens (HLA-A,B and C) are the major targets of CD8+(suppressor/cyctotoxic) lymphocytes and are expressed on the surface of mesenchymal cells of solid organs, including cardiac myocytes. The major stimuli for induction of Class-1 antigen expression is alpha and beta interferon released by activated macrophages and fibroblasts. MHC Class-2 antigens (HLA-DP, DQ and DR) are the major targets for CD4+ (inducer/help[er) lymphocytes and are expressed on the surface of endothelial cells, passenger lymphocytes, macrophages, monocytes, and dendritic cells. The major stimuli for induction of Class-2 antigen expression is gamma interferon released by activated CD4+ and CD8+ cells. The expression of MHC antigens is the rate-limiting step in the initiation of cardiac allograft rejection. *The inhibition of antigen expression will attenuate allograft rejection.*

The sequence of events in the transplant allograft response is recognition of the transplanted Class-2 antigens by the recipients own monocyte, macrophage or dendritic cells. These cells are call Antigen Presenting Cells (APC). The transplanted Class-2 antigen is absorbed by the APC, digested, reprocessed and placed on the surface of the APC in conjunction with its own Class-2 antigen (1a) as a non-covalent bond. This antigen-1a complex is necessary for recognition by the T-helper cell (CD4+). The receptor on the surface of the helper cell (TCR) recognizes the antigen-1a complex and binds it causing activation of the helper cell. It is well recognized that the helper cell requires a dual or simultaneous identification of both the antigenic determinant and a self Class-2 product (1a) in order for activation, proliferation, and induction of effector mechanisms to occur.

The helper cell is activated from a quiescent state (G-0 phase) to an actively metabolizing cell (G-1a). In the G-1a phase there is active transcription of new messenger RNA for an array of proteins that will be displayed on the cell surface as activation receptors (TCR and interleukin-1 receptor). Also there is transcription for a cytokine, interleukin-10 which stimulates macrophages. Interleukin-10 activates macrophages for the transcription of messenger RNA for de-novo synthesis of the monokine interleukin-1. The activated helper cell receives a second signal to complete its clonal expansion. This signal is provided by the binding of the Interleukin-1 from the macrophage to the new Interleukin-1 binding sites on the surface of the helper cell. The new process incorporates calcium signals as well as high energy phosphate signals in the form of ITP and the genome of the activated helper cell is stimulated to transcribe new messenger RNA for a host of cytokines such as Interleukin-2. This cytokine will serve as an autocoid (a substance made by a cell which will bind to a receptor on the surface of the same cell and alter it's function) to push it through the next two phases of the cell cycle (G1b and S). During S phase DNA is doubled and cell division occurs causing clonal expansion of the cells which are capable of responding to the given allograft.

Simultaneously with the activation of the helper pedigree of lymphocytes is the activation of the cytotoxic lymphocyte by its encounter with Class-1 antigens that are displayed on the surface of the transplant. The cytotoxic lymphocyte (CTL) does not require an APC, but binds directly to the Class-1 antigens causing activation and transcription of m-RNA. However, the CTL requires activation by T-helper cells to complete the clonal expansion event. The help is provided by the release of Interleukin-2 and other cytokines such as cytotoxic activating factor (CAF). Interleukin-2 pushes the cell through the G1b and S phases. CAF differentiates the cell into a killer cell causing lysis of the allogenic cells and the transplanted organ. CTL's produce gamma-interferon which promote recognition of Class-2 alloantigens by macrophages and perpetuates the immune response. The activated helper cells also elaborate interleukin-3 which differentiates T-cells into suppressor cells, ultimately leading to feedback suppression of the immune response.

In summary, the immune response to allograft organs consists of presentation, recognition, activation and destruction.[21-24]

IMMUNOTHERAPY

Tolerance is a non-reactive state to specific alloantigens. This state can be achieved by blocking presentation or recognition of Class-2 antigens. Ideal immunotherapy would induce specific unresponsiveness (tolerance), allow clearance of infection and tumors, and therefore, eliminate chronic therapy. Currently there is no immunosuppressive agent which induces tolerance. Presently, we utilize agents that affect immunoactivation distal to antigen presentation and recognition. As a result multiple agents in combination are required.

Steroids are commonly used agents for both chronic immunotherapy as well as rescue therapy for acute rejection. These agents inhibit interleukin-1 release by preventing transcription of messenger RNA thereby preventing interleukin-2 production and T-helper cell activation.

Azathioprine is used for chronic therapy. This agent is converted by the liver to 6-mercaptopurine and inhibits DNA and RNA synthesis in actively dividing cells. T and B cell proliferation is attenuated.

Cyclosporine is also used predominantly for chronic maintenance therapy. The mode of action of this agent is to block transcription of the interleukin-2 gene, thereby inhibiting release of cytotoxic T-cell stimulating factor, gamma interferon, and B-cell stimulating factor.

Polyclonal cytolytic agents are used for both induction therapy and for rescue therapy for acute rejection. These agents nonspecifically opsonize T-cells, inducing clearance by the reticuloendothelial system. Polyclonal antibodies against T-cell surface antigens OKT3, OKT4+, OKT8+ and OKT11+ are present in random concentrations in any given batch of sera. Examples of this type of agent are Minnesota Anti-lymphocytic Globulin (MALG) and Antithymic Globulin (ATGAM).

Monoclonal cytolytic agents are also used for induction therapy and rescue for acute rejection. OKT3 is the most commonly used monoclonal agent. This is a mouse IgG antibody directed against the CD3 surface antigen on all T-lymphocytes. The CD3 antigen forms a complex with the TCR (t-core receptor) which binds with the APC for recognition in the immune response sequence. When OKT3 binds to the CD3 antigen, it blocks the TCR and therefore prevents the recognition step of the immune response.

The particular immunotherapy regime used in any given transplant center may vary according to preference and personal experience. Most centers will use triple therapy (steroids, azathioprine and cyclosporine) or double therapy with or without cytolytic induction therapy.[25-28]

INDICATIONS FOR HEART TRANSPLANT [29,30]

a) Class 3 or 4 heart failure with prognosis for survival less than 12 months. Exercise 0_2 uptake less than 10cc/kg/min.
b) Documented myocardial ischemia with a large area at risk in a patient that is not revascularizable.
c) End stage valve disease not amenable to repair or replacement.
d) End stage congenital disease not amenable to repair.

e) Age less than 60 years.
f) Pulmonary vascular resistance less than 4 Wood units.
g) No insulin dependent diabetes mellitus.
h) No other non-reversible organ failure.
i) No systemic disease that will limit prognosis.
j) No drug or alcohol addiction, no smoking.
k) Ability to comply with a complex medical regime.
l) No active infection or recent (6 weeks) pulmonary embolus.

INDICATIONS FOR LUNG TRANSPLANT [31,32]

a) End stage pulmonary disease, oxygen-dependent with exercise incapacitation.
b) No other major organ failure - non-reversible.
c) No other limiting systemic disease.
d) No alcohol or drug dependency.
e) Emotionally stable and compliant.
f) Age less than 55 years.

PROCEDURE SELECTION

Heart-Lung Transplant

End stage pulmonary failure associated with non-reversible right heart dysfunction.

a) Primary pulmonary hypertension
b) Eisenmenger's Syndrome
c) Cystic fibrosis
d) Bronchiectasis
e) Primary idiopathic bronchiolitis
f) Alpha-1 anti-trypsin deficiency
g) Eosinophilic granulomatosis

Double Lung Transplant

End stage pulmonary failure associated with reversible right heart dysfunction. Infectious etiology.

a) Cystic fibrosis
b) Bronchiectasis
c) Eosinophilic granulomatosis

Single Lung Transplant

End stage pulmonary associated with reversible right heart dysfunction. No infectious etiology.

a) Pulmonary fibrosis
b) Emphysema
c) Primary pulmonary hypertension
d) Selected patients with Eisenmenger's syndrome and a correctable congenital heart defect (e.g., VSD)

DONOR CRITERIA[33]

a) Certified brain dead patient.
b) No arrest or prolonged hypotension.
c) Hemodynamically stable without high dose inotropes.
d) No history of cardiac or pulmonary disease.
e) No history of alcohol or drug abuse.
f) Negative serology.
g) Age less than 55 years.
h) If age greater than 40 years, require heart catheterization.
i) Normal EKG and Echo of the heart.
j) Normal CXR.
k) No thoracic trauma.
l) $PaO_2 > 300$ mmHg on FiO_2 100% or $PaO_2 > 140$ mmHg On FiO_2 40% with PEEP at 5mmHg for 30 minutes.
m) $PaCO_2 < 35$ mmHg with tidal volume 10-15 cc/kg, rate 12/min for 30 minutes.
n) Inspiratory force < 25 mmHg.
O) No fever, white blood cell count (WBC) < 10x103.

RESULTS

Heart Transplant

These data are from the International Society of Heart Transplantation registry for 1991.[34] The number of active centers peaked in 1988 near 150 and has fallen slightly in the past year. The number of procedures has peaked world wide over the past three years at 2,500. Recipient age distribution has varied from 1 day to 78 years. The majority of recipients are in the age range of 40-60 years. Over 75% of all adult transplants are male, while just over 50% of all transplants in the 18 year and under group are male. The indication for transplantation in the adult group is 50% cardiomyopathy, 40% coronary artery disease and 10% other. In the 18 year and under group still 50% of the patients had cardiomyopathy, while 40% had congenital abnormalities.

The donor age on the average has not increased over the past five years (25 years). The operative mortality increases with prolonged ischemic times doubling after 5 hours. The operative mortality also varies with age. Patients 5 years and under have an operative mortality near 25%. After 20 years it falls to 10%. The cause of mortality in the 18 year and under group is due most often to technical or cardiac reasons. In the adult population it is evenly split between rejection and infection. Survival analysis for adults shows the 1 year survival at 80% and the 5 year survival at 65%, the pediatric group has a 1 year at 70% and 5 year at 60%.

Lung Transplant

There has been a significant decrease in the number of heart-lung procedures performed over the past two years with a simultaneous rise in the number of single lung procedures. Most patients receiving heart-lung procedures are between the ages of 20-30 years. Single lung transplant is more commonly performed in the 35-55 year age group. Sixty percent of all types of lung transplants are performed in females. Operative mortality for both procedures is the same at approximately 20%. The cause of death in all groups is predominantly technical followed closely by infection. The 1 year survival for single lung transplant is 70% with a 2 year near 60%. Heart-lung has a one year survival of 60% and 2 year at 55%.

The main reason for the move to single lung transplantation over heart-lung is the significant shortage of donor organs. One donor can serve three recipients with 2 separate single lung transplants and one heart transplant versus one recipient for the heart-lung procedure.

REFERENCES

1. J.D. Hardy, C.M. Chavez, F.D. Kurrus, et al: Heart transplantation in man: Developmental studies and report of a case. *JAMA* 188:1132;1964.
2. R.R. Lower, R.C. Stofer, N.E. Shumway: Homovital transplantation in man: Developmental studies and report of a case. *J Thorac Cardiovasc Surg* 41:196;1961.
3. C.N. Barnard: A human cardiac transplant: An interim report of a successful operation performed at Groote Schur Hospital, Cape Town, *A S Med J* 41:1271;1967.
4. D.K.C. Cooper: Experimental development of cardiac transplantation. *Br Med J* 4:174;1968.
5. W.A. Baumgartner, B.A. Reitz, P.E. Oyer, et al: Cardiac homotransplantation. *Curr Probl Surg* 16:7;1979.
6. J.G. Copeland, E.B. Stinson: Human heart transplantation. *Curr Probl Cardiol* 4:1;1979.
7. M.E. Billingham, P.K. Caves, E. Dong, et al: The diagnosis of canine orthotopic cardiac allograft rejection by transvenous endomyocardia biopsy. *Transplant Proc* 1:741;1973.
8. C.P. Bieber, R.B. Griepp, P.E. Oyer, et al: Use of rabbit antithymocyte globulin in cardiac transplantation. Relationship of serum clearance rates to clinical outcome. *Transplant*, 22:478-488;1876.
9. J.G. Copeland, R.W. Emery, M.M. Levinson, et al: Cyclosporine: An immunosuppressive panacea? *J Thorac Cardiovasc Surg* 91:26;1986.
10. M.P. Kaye: The Registry of the International Society for Heart Transplantation: Fourth official report,6:63;1987.
11. A. Carrel, C.C. Guthrie: The transplantation of veins and organs. *Am Med* 10:1101;1905.

12. D.A. Cooley, R.D. Bloodwell, G.L. Hallman, et al: Organ transplantation for advanced cardiopulmonary disease. *Ann Thorac Surg* 8:30;1969.
13. B.A. Reitz, J.L. Wallwork, S.A. Hunt, et al: Heart-lung transplantation: successful therapy for patients with pulmonary vascular disease. *N Eng J Med* 306:557-64;1982.
14. H. Metras: Note preliminaire sur la greffe totale du poumon chez le chien. C R Acad Sci (Paris) 231:1176-78;1950.
15. J.D. Hardy, S. Eraslan, M.L. Dalton, et al: Lung homotransplantation in man. *JAMA* 186:1065-74;1963.
16. F. Derom, F. Barbier, S. Ringoir, et al: Ten month survival after lung homotransplantation in man. *J Thorac Surg* 61:835-46;1971.
17. J.M.W. Nelems, A.S. Rebuck, J.D. Cooper, et al: Human lung transplantation. *Chest* 78:5699-73;1980.
18. O. Lima, M. Goldberg, W.J. Peters, et al: Bronchial omentopexy in canine lung transplantation. *J Thorac Cardiovasc Surg* 83:418-21;1982.
19. The Toronto Lung Transplant Group: Experience with single lung transplantation for pulmonary fibrosis. *JAMA* 259:2258-62;1988.
20. G.A. Patterson, J.D. Cooper, B. Goldman, et al: Technique of successful clinical double-lung transplantation. *Ann Thorac Surg* 4:626-33;1988.
21. J.B. O'Connell, D.G. Renlund: Immune mechanisms of acute cardiac allograft rejection and modification by immunosuppression. *Cardiac Surgery: State of the Art Reviews* 3(3):607-611;1989.
22. D.J. Cohen, S. Joyce, L. Wetstein, et al: Basic concepts in immunobiology of organ transplantation. In *Heart Transplantation* Edited by P.D. Myerowitz, Futura Publishing Co., 19-53;1987.
23. J.H. Helderman: Mechanisms by which immunosuppressive agents prevent allograft rejection. In: *Heart and Heart-Lung Transplantation Update* Edited by V. Gallucci, U. Bortolotti, G. Faggian, and A. Mazzucco, Edizioni Scientifiche, Firenze, Italy, 3-11;1988.
24. S.J. Shumway: Basic immunologic concepts involved in organ transplantation. In: *Heart and Heart-Lung Transplantation* Edited by W.A. Baumgartner, B.A. Reitz, and S.C. Achuff. W.B. Saunders Co, Philadelphia, 15-24;1990.
25. J.B. O'Connell, D.G. Renlund, H.R. Lee, et al: Newer techniques of immunosuppression in cardiac transplantation. *Cardiac Surgery: State of the Art Reviews*, 2(4):607-615;1988.
26. R.M. Bolman, B. Elick, M.T. Olivari, et al: Improved immunosuppression for heart transplantation. *J Heart Transplant* 4:315-318;1985.
27. P.E. Oyer, E.B. Stinson, S.W. Jamieson, et al: One year experience with cyclosporine in clinical heart transplantation. *J Heart Transplant* 1:285-290;1982.
28. D.G. Renlund, J.B. O'Connell E.M. Gilbert, et al: Feasibility of discontinuation of corticosteroid maintenance therapy in heart transplantation. *J Heart Transplant* 6:71-78;1987.
29. J.G. Copeland, R.W. Emery, M.M. Levinson, et al: Selection of patients for cardiac transplantation. *Circulation* 75:2-9;1987.
30. F. Eales, R.W. Emery, L.D. Joyce, et al: Selection of heart transplant recipients and surgical techniques. In: *Cardiac Surgery: State of the Art Reviews* Vol 2, Edited by R.W. Emery, M.R. Pritzker, Hanley & Belfus, Cardiothoracic Transplantation, p 565-70;1988.
31. T.M. Egan, L.R. Kaiser, J.D. Cooper: Lung Transplantation: *Current Problems in Surgery* 26(10):681-751;1989.
32. K. Hale, M.R. Pritzker: The single lung and double lung recipient: Patient selection. In: *Cardiac Surgery: State of the Art Reviews* - Vol 2 Edited by

R.W. Emery, M.R. Pritzker; Hanley & Belfus, Cardiothoracic Transplantation, 571-574;1988.

33. F. Eales, R.W. Emery, T.J. VonRueden, et al: The cardiothoracic donor. In: *Cardiac Surgery: State of the Art Reviews* Vol 2 Edited by R.W. Emery, M.R. Pritzker; Hanley & Belfus, Cardiothoracic Transplantation, 547-54;1988.

34. J.M. Kriett, M.P. Kaye: The Registry of the International Society for Heart Transplantation: Eighth official report 10(4):491-98;1991.

CORONARY BYPASS GRAFTING IN CONJUNCTION WITH CAROTID AND VALVULAR DISEASE

Anthony J. DelRossi, M.D. and Aurel C. Cernaianu, M.D.

University of Medicine and Dentistry of New Jersey
Robert Wood Johnson Medical School at Camden
Department of Surgery, Division of Cardiothoracic Surgery
Cooper Hospital/University Medical Center
Camden, New Jersey

The intent of this chapter is to present the current status of surgical coronary revascularization in conjunction with surgery for carotid disease or valvular surgery.

CORONARY ARTERY BYPASS SURGERY COMBINED WITH CAROTID ARTERY SURGERY

Presently, there is an increased number of procedures performed on older patients with more advanced combined coronary and cerebrovascular disease. The added potential risks of concomitant cerebrovascular occlusive disease and coronary disease is of special concern[1]. In many of these patients, the carotid lesions are asymptomatic. Conversely, symptomatic coronary artery disease occurs in approximately 40% of patients undergoing carotid endarterectomy[2-4].

Recently, data from Moore et al[5] have confirmed the efficacy of surgery in preventing strokes in patients with recent hemispheric transient ischemic attacks or non-disabling strokes and in patients with ipsilateral high-grade (70%-90%) carotid stenosis.

Nevertheless, there is still controversy whether asymptomatic carotid stenosis should be regarded conservatively or operated upon. Some investigators wonder if extra-cranial revascularization should be done for non-hemispheric symptoms[6]. Since carotid endarterectomy is a prophylactic operation designed to diminish or eliminate stroke risk, its effectiveness is directly proportional to the risk of operation[7-12].

Presently, there is a consensus that symptomatic carotid artery disease may benefit from perioperative medical therapy and these patients should be treated with subsequent coronary angiography and coronary artery bypass surgery (CABG). However, the issue is controversial particularly when related to the appropriate management of the patient who requires CABG and in whom significant carotid occlusive disease is found.[13]

Stroke risk during cardiopulmonary bypass for CABG has been significantly improved from earlier experience. Recent improvements of perfusion technology have allowed a reduction in the rate of stroke during cardiopulmonary bypass (CPB). Current medical literature indicates that the risk of significant stroke during CABG is approximately 2%[14,15].

The risks factors identified by Gardner et al[16] to correlate with an increased risk of stroke during CPB include significant atherosclerotic disease of the ascending aorta, advanced age, extended ischemic time on CPB, and a prior history of cerebral vascular accident. However, these data has not been confirmed by Brener and his co-workers[17] who found an incidence of 2% central nervous system infarction during CABG but could not be predicted by any of the perioperative variables.

The pathology of stroke during CPB has been related to the formation of microemboli from the ascending aorta and the left ventricle and microaggregation of platelets and gaseous microemboli from the oxygenator[15]. Bone wax and fat particles may also be implicated. Also, watershed infarctions from cerebral high flow perfusion do occur as evidenced by the high stroke risk of 14% reported by Brener and coworkers[17] in patients with chronic internal carotid artery occlusion. Although cerebral perfusion may increase during non-pulsatile CPB, these data come from studies performed in patients without significant carotid occlusive disease[18], demonstrating that stroke during CPB for CABG is multifactorial.

The effect of concomitant coronary artery disease and its major contribution to short and long-term mortality in patients requiring carotid endarterectomy has been described by Hertzer et al[19]. Moreover, Hertzer et al[14], and Brener et al[17], demonstrated that severe carotid stenosis greater than 70% occurs in less than 4% in patients undergoing elective surgical coronary revascularization. Experience from Massachusetts General Hospital shows that less than 2% of all CABG patients are to be considered for combined procedures. Again, it is difficult to assess the effect of CPB to stroke, particularly because the two entities, i.e. the coronary artery disease and carotid artery disease may have a low combined incidence. Indeed, the centrifugal bypass circuit itself causes blood surface interaction. The pump apparatus (roller occlusive versus centrifugal) or pulsatile versus nonpulsatile has a measurable effect upon cerebral perfusion.

Data from Breslau et al[20] and Barnes et al[21] did not find that carotid disease is an important risk factor for stroke during cardiovascular operations. The authors of these studies have demonstrated that there is a poor relationship between carotid bruit and the anatomic lesion. However, these studies did not address many issues related to carotid disease and the risk of stroke during CPB, including patients at questionable risk, or patients with asymptomatic bruits, and questionable severity of carotid disease (50% or greater diameter stenosis).

Recent data[14] from a randomized prospective study of patients undergoing concomitant carotid and surgical myocardial revascularization have clearly demonstrated that there is an association between the presence of advanced carotid occlusive disease and the incidence of stroke.

The risk of stroke or transient ischemic attack (TIA), in patients with asymptomatic carotid disease who underwent CABG has been found to be significantly higher than in those without carotid artery disease (9.2% versus 1.9%, $p < 0.05$)[17].

In the CABG patient, the risk of stroke or TIA is increased also by the presence of carotid bruit (3.9 fold), prior history of stroke, extended ischemic time during CPB, and advanced patient age [22]. These results have been confirmed by other large published series[14,17].

If the concept that severe carotid stenosis may increase the risk of perioperative stroke in small percentage of CABG patients with concomitant disease, then, the important question is if this risk may be the same if the surgery is performed as a staged or simultaneous carotid endarterectomy. The short-term goal is protection from stroke during cardiopulmonary bypass, however, there are other consequences of severe carotid stenosis in terms of perioperative stroke risk in the patient undergoing CABG. A number of technical algorithms have been developed for the patient who requires treatment of both lesions. Carotid endarterectomy followed by CABG represents the "staged" procedure. Simultaneous operation with endarterectomy performed immediately prior to the institution of CPB and the so-called "reverse-staged" approach where CABG is performed first followed by elective carotid surgery at some interval thereafter are also possible alternatives. Each technique has its theoretical potential advantages and disadvantages. Staged carotid endarterectomy may increase the time of cardiac ischemia as a complication of the carotid operation. Since the carotid lesion remains initially uncorrected, the reverse-staged approach where myocardial revascularization takes places first, increases the risk of perioperative stroke. Simultaneous operations while appealing in theory have been accompanied by increased morbidity in many reports[13].

Perioperative complications for isolated carotid endarterectomy (CEA) and combined coronary and carotid surgery are shown in Table 1 (reproduced with permission from Cambria RP, Brewster DC. Coexisting Coronary and Carotid Disease; Combined or Staged Operation?. Semin Vasc Surg 1989;2:43-49). These data represents the reported cumulative experience in the literature from approximately 30 series including those from Massachusetts General Hospital related to com-

Table 1

Operation	No. of Patients	Mortality (%)	MI (%)	Stroke (%)
CEA (MGH 1986-1987)	203	0.5	2.0	1.0
CABG (MGH 1983-1987)	3570	2.2	1.2	0.6
CEA/CABG (MGH 1983-1987)	51	2.0	0	2.0
CEA/CABG (Collective)*	1515	5.6	3.8	3.1

bined carotid endarterectomy and CABG. The surveyed collective average mortality was 5.6% and the presence of stroke with permanent deficit was 3.1 %. These data presents mortality rates which are higher then the mortality rate of a controlled population undergoing isolated CABG, probably because patients undergoing the combined operation may present with more advanced cardiac disease than their counterparts presenting for CABG without carotid disease.

Table 2 (reproduced with permission from Cambria RP, Brewster DC. Coexisting Coronary and Carotid disease; Combined or Staged Operation?. Semin Vasc Surg 1989;2:43-49) presents data from the Massachusetts General Hospital study comparing patients undergoing isolated CABG and those who have undergone the combined procedure. Patients undergoing simultaneous operation had significantly more left main coronary disease, as well as signs of more advanced left ventricular dysfunction. In consequence, approximately 20% of the patients undergoing combined procedures required cardiac assistance with intra-aortic balloon pump for either, unstable preoperative angina or for weaning from CPB. As mentioned before, the overall risk of surgery in patients with combined lesion may be higher as a function of more advanced cardiac disease. According to Cambria and Brewster[13], "patients who require treatment of both lesions will undergo combined operation on the basis of the severity of the coronary artery disease. In such patients, the risk of proceeding with an initial staged carotid operation seems inappropriate since the results do not document increased risks in proceeding with a combined CEA/CABG approach".

Despite favorable series presented in Table 1, the combined procedure presents with some disadvantages. Prolonging an already major surgical procedure, the complexity of EEG monitoring, and the involvement of the surgical procedure, are some of the major concerns related

Table 2

	CABG	CEA/CABG
No. of patients	1,038*	71†
M/F Ratio	4/1	4/1
Age (mean yr)	62.6	65.2
Duration CPB (min)	91.3	95.1
No. of CABG (mean)	4.0	3.8
Unstable angina (%)	48%	68%
Left Main CAD	9.8%‡	37%‡

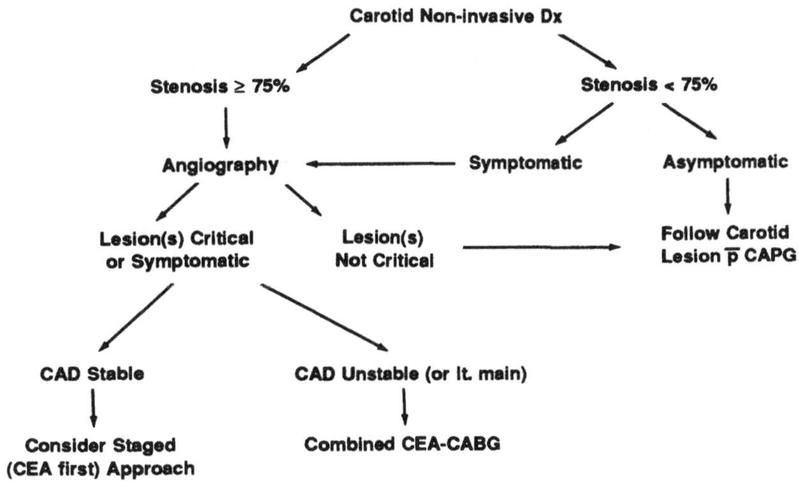

Figure 1

to this procedure. Decreasing the operative time by performing the vein harvest during the initial CEA, or operating without EEG monitoring, (however, with shunting) may resolve some of these problems. Furthermore, since the operative outcome is dependent on the speed of achieving the carotid operation, these surgical procedures are inadequate for being performed by residents and/or fellows. The anesthetic and blood pressure requirements for carotid and coronary disease may be in conflict. Anesthesia for the CABG allows the patients to be asleep for 6 to 12 hours postoperatively; this will make the early assessments of the patient's neurologic status quite difficult.

According to Cambria et al[13], the most important factor in deciding between staged versus combined operations is the stability of the coronary artery disease. Unstable angina, intra-aortic balloon support and significant coronary artery disease are determinant factors for an initial staged carotid endarterectomy. However, with appropriate expert anesthetic management, patients with stable coronary artery disease, may have a safe and successful carotid operation.

Carotid endarterectomy might be performed under local anesthesia in a specific category of patients as part of the overall strategy towards staged treatment of the lesions.

The merits of the various combinations of surgical staging in patients with coexisting carotid and coronary disease has been reported by Hertzer et al[14]. This randomized, prospective study included 275 patients (approximately 3% of total CABG experience during that time interval). undergoing carotid operations with either symptomatic and/or severe, greater than 70% diameter carotid stenosis. Ten percent of these patients had unstable coronary artery disease and contraindications for an initial staged carotid operation. One hundred twenty-nine patients with unilateral, asymptomatic, severe, carotid stenosis were randomized to either combined operation, or reverse-staged. The mortality rate for the patients undergoing the combined operation was

4.2 %, and was associated with a stroke rate of 2.8%. The reverse-staged CEA-treated patients had an incidence of perioperative stroke of 14%. Also, the risk of stroke with the CABG alone and an uncorrected carotid lesion was 6.9%.

The anatomic location of carotid endarterectomy has not been found to be a good predictor of stroke in patients undergoing the combined procedure[14]. The authors rather have attributed these results to hemodynamically mediated cerebral infarction or diffuse atheroembolization. It can be concluded that the presence of significant carotid artery disease may increase the risk of stroke in patients undergoing CABG proportionally to its severity and the presence or absence of clinical symptoms.

The results presented here suggest that the performance of CEA should be delayed in the early phase post CABG. The patient management should be dictated by the degree of the coronary artery disease i.e., patients with stable coronary artery disease may undergo a safe initial staged carotid endarterectomy. If the status of the coronary artery disease is such that initial stage operation is unsafe, then combined operation is logical[23].

Figure 1 (reproduced with permission from Cambria RP, Brewster DC. Coexisting Coronary and Carotid disease; Combined or Staged Operation?. Semin Vasc Surg 1989;2:43-49) is a tentative algorithm of a patient with combined carotid and coronary artery disease showing that carotid lesions should be corrected on their own merit prior to CABG if the patient is hemodynamically stable. Since this situation is the exception rather than common, the combined CEA/CABG approach represent the best alternative.

In summary, the patients with combined carotid and coronary artery disease may present with different degrees of severity of disease. This in turn, points to a variety of solutions for patient management. The surgical technique should be individualized. Asymptomatic carotid disease needs surgical treatment if the stenotic lesions is greater than 80% are found. In addition, clinical status, particularly the stability of the coronary artery disease represents the principal criteria for selecting the most adequate patient management when the two lesions are present.

CORONARY ARTERY BYPASS GRAFTING AND VALVULAR DISEASE

Patients undergoing valvular heart surgery often present with concomitant coronary artery disease in up to 48% of all cases[24-27]. Data compiled by Winters and Samuels[28] has proven that combined surgery for patients with valvular and coronary disease has a low operative risk and favorable long-term outcome. The concomitant performance of CABG and cardiac valve surgery raises some issues related to the detrimental as well as the beneficial effect of the combined procedure.

Randomized studies assessing the benefit of surgical myocardial revascularization in patients requiring valve operation with coexistent significant symptomatic coronary artery disease are very difficult to implement particularly if an improved quality of life or increased survival time are the end points. However, data demonstrating that patients undergoing the combined procedure have neither an increased risk of surgery, nor a decreased long-term survival would provide the support for the rationale of such procedure.

The increased use of coronary angiography in patients with valvular heart disease, particularly in those with an increased age, results in a higher chance for diagnosis of coexisting coronary arteriosclerosis and valvular disease. Myocardial revascularization has been proven as an effective and safe modality of treatment for patients with significant coronary artery disease, and isolated elective CABG has a low operative mortality rate of 1 to 3%. Although myocardial revascularization combined with valve replacement has become standard at most medical centers, this kind of operation is still controversial. Different series have presented inconsistent results. Differences in the etiology of the valvular disease, the type of valve prosthesis used, the perioperative functional and hemodynamic status, age, and the severity of the coronary artery disease, have all been found to be predictors of outcome for such procedures[25]. High operative mortality rates have been reported for specific subpopulations of patients. Some patients with mitral regurgitation and coronary artery disease may have a better result with revascularization alone. On the other hand, patients with combined aortic stenosis and coronary artery disease may have a better result when they undergo aortic valve replacement with myocardial revascularization.

The list of potential risks factors includes advanced age, reoperation, requirement of extensive revascularization, and severe left ventricular dysfunction. Each of these factors add approximately 6% to the surgical mortality. In the presence of an ejection fraction less than 20% or global hypokinesia, the mortality risk doubles.

MITRAL VALVE SURGERY COMBINED WITH CABG

When mitral regurgitation is associated with coronary artery disease it may be difficult to assess the components of each disease. Some objective criteria have been defined to quantify the degree of mitral regurgitation such as murmur, findings of the chest roentgenogram , echocardiography, angiocardiography and left ventriculography, and the intraoperative findings.

It is important to emphasize that mitral valve dysfunction may result from myocardial ischemia which may change the indications for and results of surgery when the combination of these two conditions co-exist.

Acute, severe mitral regurgitation is characterized by a murmur which tends to decrease in intensity or be absent in late systole with an occasional crescendo-decrescendo configuration. Different degrees of papillary muscle dysfunction may translate in a mid-systolic, late systolic, or even early systolic murmur. Approximately 50% of the patients may present with a systolic murmur of mitral regurgitation during or recovering from myocardial infarction[29] and its intensity depends upon the extent of myocardia ischemia. The murmur may be audible only in the presence of angina. Its degree of intensity may depend on the patient's hydration status and may be exacerbated with ST-T wave changes.

Chest roentgenogram findings should corroborate with the hemodynamic status. Systolic or diastolic left ventricular dysfunction may cause pulmonary hypertension. Ischemic mitral regurgitation is characterized by a small or only mildly enlarged left atrium.

Mitral regurgitation of ischemic origin may be graded as mild, moderate, or severe. Its severity depends upon the patient's state of hydration, left ventricular function, the presence or absence of arrhythmia, and the degree of myocardial ischemia. During the angiographic assessment, the position of the left ventricular catheter may induce false positive or false negative results if its placement is incorrect.

The sensitivity and specificity of echocardiographic techniques with color Doppler have been found to correlate with the angiocardiographic degree of mitral regurgitation[30]. The Doppler should be used in a serial

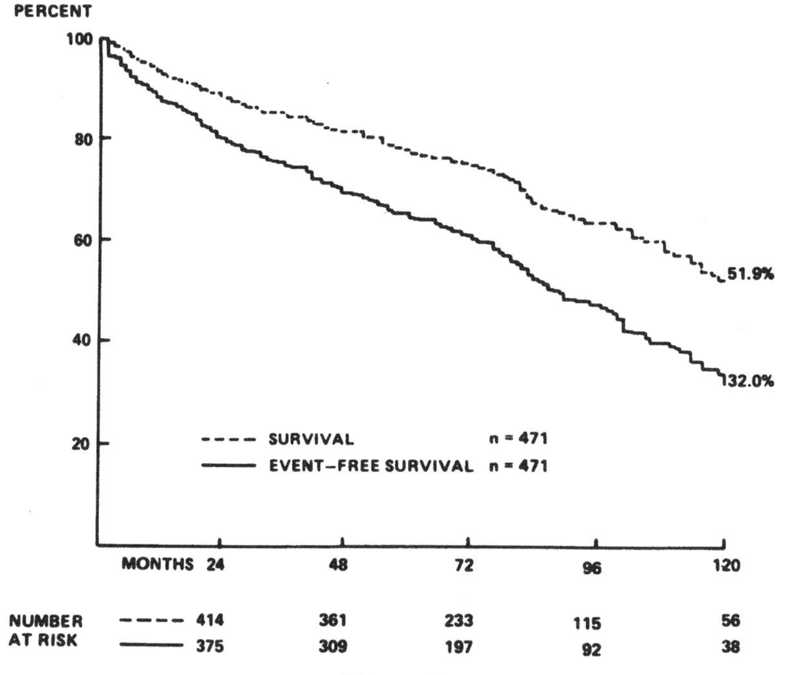

Figure 2

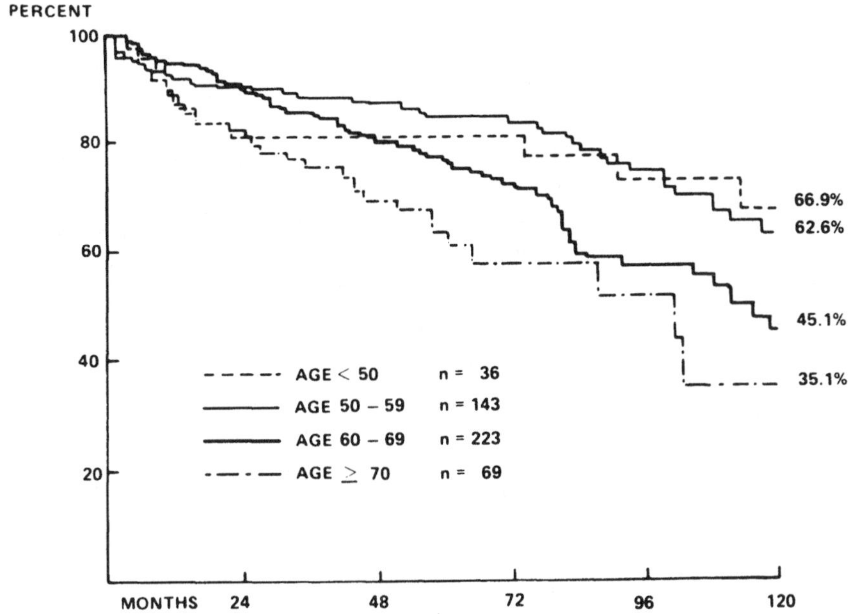

NUMBER AT RISK	24	48	72	96	120
- - - -	29	29	26	15	10
———	129	119	86	54	28
━━━	200	160	105	39	17
- — - —	56	45	16	7	1

Figure 3

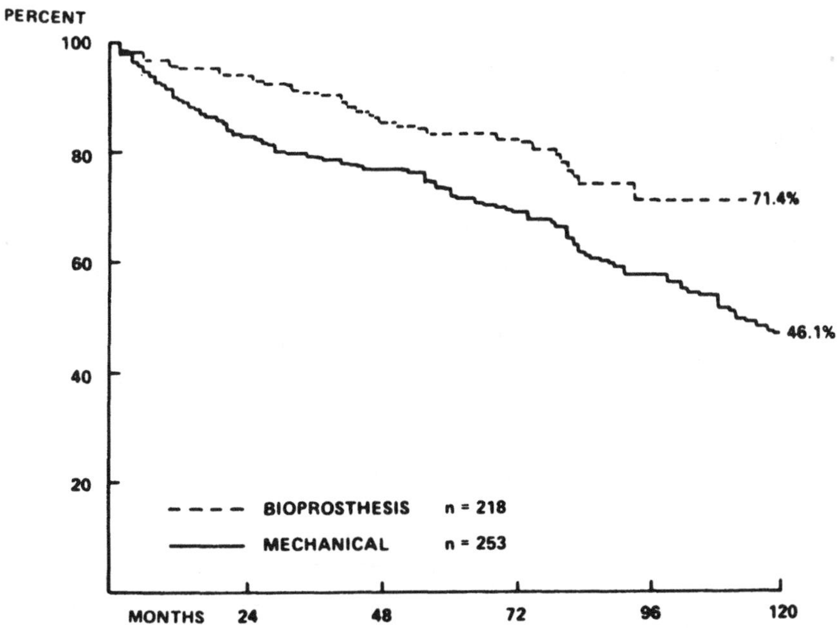

NUMBER AT RISK	24	48	72	96	120
- - - -	204	172	91	23	0
———	210	189	142	92	56

Figure 4

fashion to estimate the presence and the severity of mitral valve dysfunction. A single Doppler examination may not be sufficient to establish the final picture. We should mention however, that newer techniques like transesophageal echocardiography (TEE), are finding their way in the intraoperative arsenal for the assessment of valvular disease.

The intraoperative assessment of the regurgitant jet can be performed prior to CPB by palpating posteriorly, behind the inferior vena cava and anteriorly at the roof of the left atrium below the root of the aorta[31]. An anterior regurgitant bruit indicates a lesion located on the posterior leaflet. Conversely, a posterior jet should raise questions about an anterior incompetent leaflet. Pulmonary artery occlusion pressure (PAOP), or the left atrial pressure may add to the clinical picture. Visualization of the mitral valve should not be the only criteria for determining the degree of mitral dysfunction since the presence of mitral incompetence may be only confirmed, but its severity cannot be precisely assessed.

It is important to re-emphasize that an assessment of the degree of mitral valve incompetence based on a single examination may not be accurate in the presence of ischemic myocardial disease. Serial examination using both, clinical and diagnostic criteria may help in establishing the severity of mitral valve disease.

As a rule, the severity of mitral regurgitation may decrease over time. Some exceptions apply particularly when there is papillary muscle scarring or rupture of the chordal system. In the case of papillary muscle rupture, emergency surgical repair may be indicated in the first 6 to 8 hours.

The clinical picture of mitral regurgitation of ischemic origin resembles that of cardiomyopathy. It carries a poorer prognosis than the isolated mitral regurgitation of other origin. As mentioned previously, the outcome of mitral regurgitation of ischemic origin is correlated with the severity of left ventricular dysfunction and to the severity of mitral regurgitation.

Data presented by Balu and co-workers[32] examined the outcome of 104 patients with mitral regurgitation and coronary artery disease treated either medically or surgically. At 18.5 months follow-up, survival rate in the surgical group was 90 % which was significantly different from those treated medically (57.5%). This demonstrated that approximately 40 % of the patients with mitral valve regurgitation of ischemic origin may die in the first 24 months if myocardial revascularization is not performed.

The new line of thought is that the mitral valve should be repaired more frequently than being replaced[33,34]. There is information that left ventricular function is preserved when repair is done, compared with replacement[35]. The functional assessment of the mitral valve is imperfect with the use of current diagnostic techniques to determine correctly the cause of mitral valve incompetence. In consequence, the decision

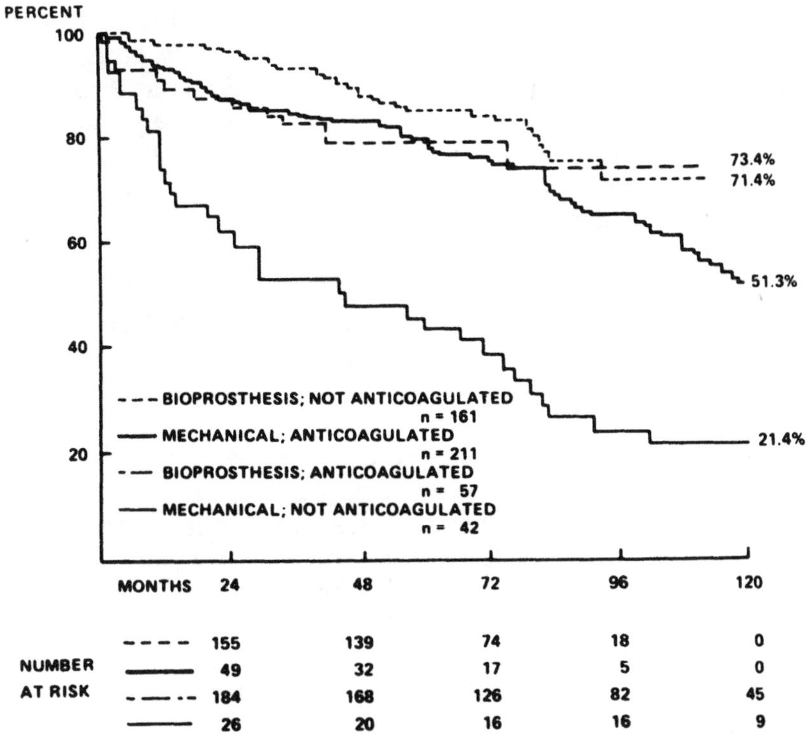

Figure 5

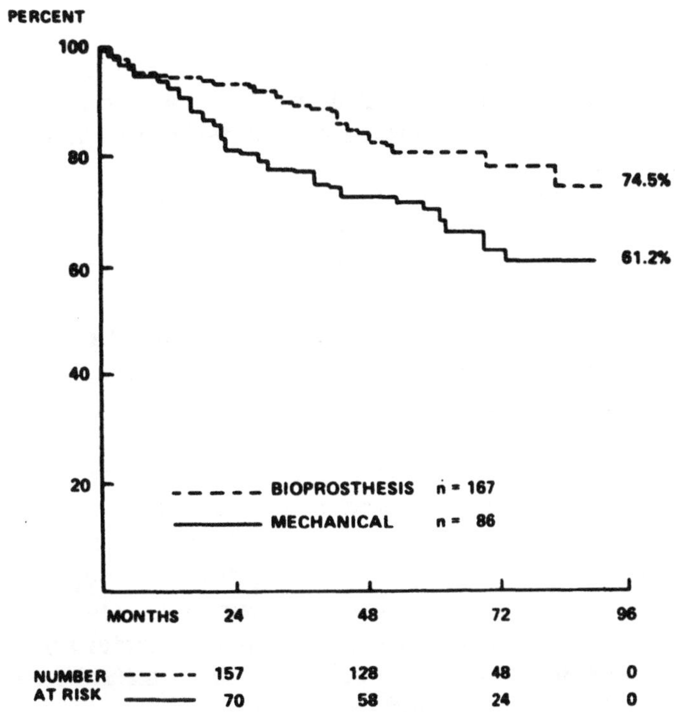

Figure 6

of which the best reparative procedure may be difficult. Generally, valve replacement has a better chance for creating a competent valve, particularly in the presence of left ventricular dysfunction.

Although the concept of mitral valve repair for valve incompetence of ischemic origin is gaining support, some authors[31] have criticized the published results because not all the cases came from procedures done on ischemic mitral valve disease or from operations done in patients with poor left ventricular function.

Kay and co-workers[36] presented data from 141 patients with mitral valve incompetence of ischemic origin who underwent either repair, or replacement. Patients undergoing mitral valve repair had an improved short-, and long-term survival rate than those patients undergoing valve replacement.

There is a consensus that only patients with severe mitral regurgitation should undergo valve repair or replacement. The decision making process should take into consideration the intensity of regurgitation, the degree of coronary ischemia, the wall motion score, ejection fraction and remoteness of infarction among others.

The effect of the severity of mitral valve regurgitation on the operative mortality has been studied by Pinson et al [37]. The authors have shown that long-term survival was related to the severity of mitral regurgitation.

Additionally, severe paradoxic segmental wall dysfunction has been found to significantly influence the survival.

Mitral regurgitation of ischemic origin is associated with a worse operative and long-term survival. Salomon and co-workers[38] from Stanford demonstrated that the primary cause of mitral valve disease had a significant influence on long-term survival, i.e., the mitral valve dysfunction of rheumatic, myxomatous, or ischemic origin has different long-term outcome.

The probability of survival after mitral valve replacement in patients with coronary artery disease has been presented by Chaffin and Daggett[39]. The authors have shown that untreated myocardial ischemia represents a major risk factor for death after mitral valve replacement because ischemia may produce ventricular dilatation and papillary muscle dysfunction resulting in scarring or fiber lengthening, or annular dilatation, chordal stretch, rupture or prolapse.

When one wants to establish the operative risk score for patients undergoing concomitant valve surgery and CABG, one should consider the etiology of coronary artery disease, the wall motion abnormalities, left ventricular performance, the degree of pulmonary hypertension, and patient's age. In addition, long-term survival depends upon the performance of myocardial revascularization. Leaving coronary artery disease untreated, increases mortality. Coronary artery disease particularly ischemic cardiomyopathy accompanied by mitral regurgitation is associated with a worse long-term prognosis.

The definition of an ischemic mitral valve lesion has been described by Kay and his associates[36], who found in all cases a uniform annular

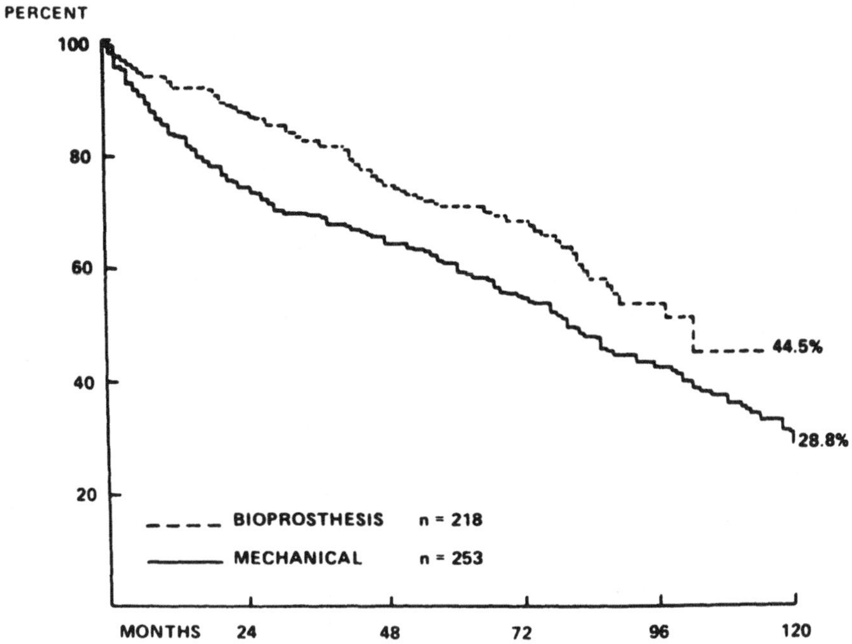

NUMBER AT RISK	24	48	72	96	120
- - - - -	188	150	82	21	0
———	187	159	115	71	38

Figure 7

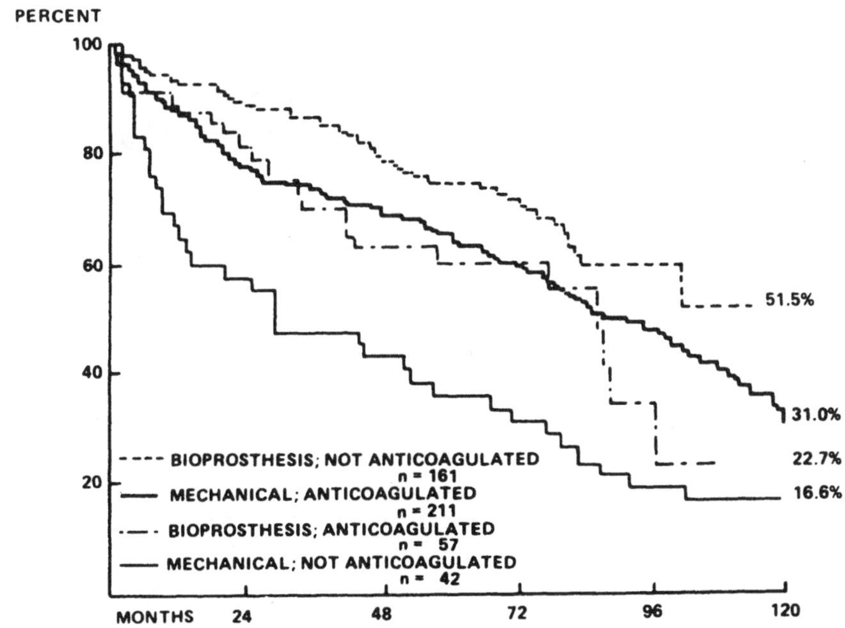

NUMBER AT RISK	24	48	72	96	120
- - - - -	143	124	68	18	0
▬▬▬	163	141	102	63	32
— · — · —	45	26	14	3	0
———	24	18	13	8	7

Figure 8

dilatation. These authors also found that mitral regurgitation of ischemic origin is characterized by the evidence of myocardial infarction antedating the murmur of mitral regurgitation, no evidence of any connective tissue disorder, intra-operative evidence of papillary muscle ischemia and lack of intraoperative findings of mitral valve prolapse, commissural fusion or other stigmata of inflammatory valve disease.

The management plan for a patient with mitral regurgitation and coronary artery disease should be individualized. Generally, papillary muscle rupture requires emergency operation. CABG and mitral valve replacement is necessary in order to allow the patient any chance of survival. In all other situations, stabilization of the ventricular function and temporization of the operative intervention should be applied. Left ventricular support with intra-aortic balloon pumping may be warranted. With such treatment, the mitral regurgitation will eventually improve. Serial measurements by color Doppler echocardiography and frequent clinical auscultation are warranted. The delayed approach may permit an improvement in the patient's cardiac function, increasing the chances of survival. However, some patients will need earlier intervention. In the case of severe mitral regurgitation, approximately 60% of the patients will undergo mitral valve replacement. In the remaining 40%, valve repair with a Carpentier ring annuloplasty or a bicommissural annuloplasty will be performed[36]. Repeated doses of oxygenated blood potassium cardioplegia are usually used. In the instances where the operation should be implemented fast, a minimum of coronary bypasses should be performed, since "complete" revascularization is not warranted.

The results of the combined operation have been analyzed by investigators from Cleveland Clinic[40]. A 7.3% mortality rate has not improved over time. The same kind of data has been produced by other investigators[41,42], although many improvements related to myocardial protection have been applied over time. In consequence, an operative mortality rate between 7% and 20% and 50% to 60% survival rate at 5 years should be expected.

The strategies that might decrease the operative risk have been listed by Karp[31]. Among general and specific items are aggressive hemodynamic support before operation, pharmacologic and mechanical unloading and vigorous inotropic interventions, the establishment of a policy of extended observation before operation (if patient's status permits), a determined effort to avoid mitral surgery except in severe regurgitation, a closer look at repair as opposed to valve replacement and finally an extended control of reperfusion following removal of the aortic cross clamp.

Improvement of the postoperative outcome should remain a challenge for the operating surgeon by increasing peripheral circulation, cardiac output and an improvement of oxygen transport parameters. Only this way, the results of the surgical treatment of mitral valve disease and coronary artery disease may be optimized with resultant improved survival rate.

MYOCARDIAL REVASCULARIZATION AND AORTIC VALVE REPLACEMENT

Aortic valve stenosis and coronary artery disease can independently cause myocardial ischemia resulting in angina, myocardial infarction and death. Patients with symptomatic aortic stenosis have a poor long-term survival rate without surgery regardless if they present with coronary artery disease or not[43]. Moreover, isolated coronary artery disease decreases patient survival[44].

With an increase in the use of coronary arteriography in patients examined for valvular heart disease, the coexistence of aortic valve disease and significant coronary atherosclerosis has been found to be between 20% and 50%[45]. Of this group of patients having both diseases, 20 to 30% develop angina pectoris.

Magovern and his associates[46] and Kirklin et al[47] analyzed the risk factors for early and late death in patients undergoing combined aortic valve replacement and CABG. They found that the advanced age, emergency operation, PAOC greater than 18 mmHg, a cardiac index less than 2 $l/min/mm^2$ and a mean pulmonary artery pressure greater than 30 mmHg are predictors of early mortality when analyzed by univariant analysis. The authors have also shown that elements such as preoperative age, male sex, left ventricular end-diastolic pressure, functional class and cardiac index correlate with an increased late mortality.

The presence of left ventricular hypertrophy and coronary stenosis presents special problems in achieving optimal myocardial perfection. Myocardial protection and combined aortic valve replacement and myocardial revascularization presents special problems. When cold blood cardioplegia is used for myocardial protection, myocardial injuries such as perioperative infarction and cardiogenic shock requiring intra-aortic balloon counterpulsation or inotropic support are seen in a lesser proportion. Lytle et al[48] showed that the hospital mortality rate decreased from 5.8% to 3.4% when the use of cold potassium cardioplegia became routine.

Generally, results of aortic valve replacement and myocardial revascularization are discussed in terms of survival, early and late-term survival, event-free survival, the magnitude of postoperative symptoms and the status postoperative graft patency.

Figure 2 (from Lytle BW et al[48], reproduced by permission) presents data from a recent study published by a group from Cleveland Clinic from 500 consecutive patients undergoing concomitant aortic valve replacement and CABG. This diagram shows late- survival and event-free survival curve for 471 in-hospital survivors of aortic valve replacement combined with coronary bypass grafting. Survival rates were

88%, 81%, 74%, 63%, and 52%, and event-free survival rates were 80%, 69%, 60%, 48% and 32% at 2, 4, 6, 8, and 10 postoperative years respectively.

Figure 3 (from Lytle BW et al[48], reproduced by permission) is a diagram showing late-survival curves for in-hospital survivors for aortic valve replacement combined with coronary bypass grafting according to decade of life. Survival rates from patients younger than 50 years, 50-59 years, 60-69 years, and 70 years of age or older at operation were 81, 84, 76% and 63% at five years and 73%, 74%, 57%, and 51% at 8 year postoperatively, respectively.

Figure 4 (from Lytle BW et al[48], reproduced by permission) is a diagram of late-survival curves for in hospital survivors of aortic valve replacement combined with coronary artery bypass grafting according to aortic valve prosthesis type. Survival rate at 2, 5, and 8 postoperative years were 94 %, 83%, and 71% for patients with biologic prosthesis and 83%, 73% and 57% for patients with mechanical valves respectively.

Figure 5 (from Lytle BW et al[48], reproduced by permission) is a diagram showing late-survival curves for aortic valve replacement combined with coronary bypass grafting according to valve-anticoagulant group. For patients with prior prosthesis, survival rate at 2, 5, and 8 years were 96% 85%, and 71%, respectively, if they did not receive warfarin and 88%, 79%, and 73% if they did. For patients with mechanical prosthesis, survival rate at 2, 5, and 8 years were 62%, 43% and 24% if they did not receive warfarin and 87%, 79% and 65% if they did.

Figure 6 (from Lytle BW et al[48], reproduced by permission) is a diagram showing late-survival curves of aortic valve replacement combined with coronary bypass grafting according to prosthesis type. Survival rates at 4 and 6 postoperative years were 84% and 81%, respectively for patients with bioprosthesis and 73% and 64% for patients with mechanical prosthesis.

Figure 7 (from Lytle BW et al[48], reproduced by permission) is a diagram showing late event-free survival curves for in-hospital survivors of aortic valve replacement combined with bypass grafting according to prosthesis type. Event-free survival rate were 87%, 70%, and 53% at 2.2, 5, and 8 postoperative years, respectively for patients with bioprosthesis and 74%, 60% and 42% for patients with mechanical prosthesis.

Figure 8 (from Lytle BW et al[48], reproduced by permission) is a diagram showing late event-free survival curves for in-hospital survivors for aortic valve replacement combined with bypass grafting according to prosthesis anticoagulation group. Event-free survival rates for patients with bioprosthesis were 89%, 74%, and 59% at 2, 5, and 8 postoperative years respectively without warfarin and 80%, 60%, and 34% with warfarin.

In conclusion, this review demonstrates that presently there is sufficient data in the literature to suggest that surgical myocardial revascularization, even in those patients with single vessel coronary artery disease is warranted in view of the increased myocardial oxygen demand due to hypertrophy of the left ventricle when aortic stenosis is present. CABG as an ancillary procedure does not increase the risk of postoperative death or perioperative myocardial infarction and certainly does not jeopardize the long-term survival. With the selection of a suitable valve substitute, concomitant CABG and aortic valve surgery will result in normal hemodynamics.

REFERENCES

1. F.D. Loop: Changing management of carotid stenosis in coronary artery surgery patients (editorial) *Ann Thorac Surg* 45(6):591-592;1988.
2. M. Hennerici, A. Avlich, W. Sandmann, H.J. Freund: Incidence of asymptomatic extracranial arterial disease. *Stroke* 12:750;1981.
3. B.J. Brenner, D.K. Brief, J. Alpert, et al: A four-year experience with preoperative noninvasive carotid evaluation of two thousand twenty-six patients undergoing cardiac surgery. *J Vasc Surg* 1:326;1984.
4. G.M. Lawrie, G.C. Morris: Combined coronary and carotid revascularization. In: *Modern technics in surgery: Cardiothoracic Surgery.* Edited by L.H. Cohn, New York, Futura Publishing Co. Inc. 1:1-21;1980.
5. D.J. Moore, M.P. Sheehan, P. Kolm, et al: Are strokes predictable with noninvasive methods: A five year follow-up of 303 unoperated patients. *J Vasc Surg* 2:654-660;1985.
6. W.J. Quinones-Baedich: Asymptomatic carotid stenosis: observe, operate or both? *Sem Vasc Surg* 2:4-11;1989.
7. E.L. Jones: Combined carotid and coronary surgery - when is it necessary. *J Cardiovasc Med* 8:676-80;1983.
8. N.R. Hertzer, F.D. Loop, P.C. Taylor, E.G. Beven: Staged and combined surgical approach to simultaneous carotid and coronary vascular disease. *Surgery* 84:803-11;1978.
9. F.L. Korompoi, R.H. Hayward, W.L. Knight: Non-cardiac operations combined with coronary artery bypass. *Surg Clin North Am* 62:215-24;1982.
10. J.E. Okies, Q. MacManus, A. Starr: Myocardial revascularization and carotid endarterectomy: Combined approach. *Ann Thorac Surg* 23:560-3;1979.
11. H.C. Urschel, M.A. Razzuk, M.A. Gardner: Management of concomitant occlusive disease of the carotid and coronary arteries. *J Thorac Cardiovasc Surg* 72:829-34;1976.
12. J. Mannick: When to combine bypass with carotid endarterectomy. *J Cardiovasc Med* 8:629-32;1983.
13. R.P. Cambria, D.C. Brewster: Coexisting Coronary and carotid disease: Combined or staged procedure? *Sem Vasc Surg* 2:43-48;1989.
14. N.R. Hertzer, F.D. Loop, E.G. Beven, et al: Surgical staging for synchronous coronary and carotid disease: A study including prospective randomization. *J Vasc Surg* 9:455-63;1989.
15. T.D. Ivey: Combined carotid and coronary disease - A conservative strategy. *J Vasc Surg* 3:687-689;1986.
16. T.J. Gardner, P.J. Horneffer, T.A. Manolio, et al: Major stroke after coronary artery bypass surgery. Changing magnitude of the problem. *J Vasc Surg* 3:684-94;1986.
17. B.J. Brener, D.K. Brief, J. Alprt, et al: The risk of stroke in patients with asymptomatic carotid stenosis undergoing cardiac surgery. A follow-up study. *J Vasc Surg* 5:269-277;1987.

18. T. Lundar, K.F. Lindegaard, T. Froysaker, et al: Cerebral perfusion during nonpulsatile cardiopulmonary bypass. *Ann Thorac Surg* 40:144-150;1985.
19. N.R. Hertzer, C.D. Lees: Fatal myocardial infarction following carotid endarterectomy. Three hundred thirty-five patients followed 6-11 years after operation. *Ann Surg* 194:212-218;1981.
20. P.J. Breslau, G. Fell, T.D. Ivey, et al: Carotid arterial disease in patients undergoing coronary artery bypass operations. *J Thorac Cardiovasc Surg* 82:765-67;1981.
21. R.W. Barnes, P.B. Marszalek: Asymptomatic carotid disease in the cardiovascular surgical patient. Is Prophylactic Endarterectomy necessary? *Stroke* 12:497-500;1981.
22. G.L. Reed, D.E. Singer, E.H. Picard, et al: Stroke following coronary artery bypass surgery: a case-control estimate of the risk of carotid bruits. N Engl J Med 319:1246-1250;1988.
23. R.P. Cambria, B.L. Ivarsson, C.W. Akins, et al: Simultaneous carotid and coronary disease: Safety of the combined approach. *J Vasc Surg* 9:56-64;1989.
24. H.R. Phillips, R.H. Levine, J.E. Carter, et al: Mitral valve replacement for isolated mitral regurgitation: Analysis of clinical course and late postoperative left ventricular ejection fraction. *Am J Cardiol* 48:647;1981.
25. L.S.C. Czer, R.J. Gray, M.A. DeRobertis, et al: Mitral valve replacement: Impact of coronary artery disease and determinants of prognosis after revascularization. *Circulation* 70:1-19;1984.
26. D.C. Miller, E.B. Stinson, S.J. Rossiter, et al: Impact of simultaneous myocardial revascularization on operative risk, functional result, and survival following mitral valve replacement. *Surgery* 84:848;1978.
27. Aortic valve replacement combined with myocardial revascularization. *J Thorac Cardiovasc Surg* 95:402-14;1988.
28. W.L. Winters, D.A. Samuels: Long-term prognosis following valvular heart surgery. *Cardiovasc Clin* 16:437-505;1986.
29. F. Helmcke, N.C. Nanda, M.C. Hsiung, et al: Color Doppler assessment of mitral regurgitation with orthogonal planes. *Circulation* 75:175-183;1987.
30. J. Heikkila: Mitral incompetence complication acute myocardial infarction. *Br Heart J* 29:162-69;1967.
31. R.B. Karp, Special considerations in mitral valve and coronary artery disease. Edited by R.B. K, N.T. Kouchoukos, H. Laks, A.S. Wechsler, Year Book Medical Publishers, Inc., Chicago,p 77-92;1990.
32. V. Balu, S. Hershowitz, A.R.Z. Masud, et al: Mitral regurgitation in coronary artery disease. *Chest* 81:550-55;1982.
33. A. Carpentier: Cardiac valve surgery: The "French correction." *J Thorac Cardiovasc Surg* 86:323-37;1983.
34. C.G. Duran, J.L. Pomar, J.M. Revuelta, et al: Conservative operation for mitral insufficiency: Critical analysis supported by postoperative hemodynamic studies of 72 patients. *J Thorac Cardiovasc Surg* 79:326-337;1980.
35. L.I. Bonchek, G.N. Olinger, R. Siegel, et al: Left ventricular performance after mitral reconstruction for mitral regurgitation. *J Thorac Cardiovasc Surg* 88:122-127;984.
36. G.L. Kay, J.H. Kay, P. Zubiate et al: Mitral valve repair for mitral regurgitation secondary to coronary artery diseases. *Circulation* 74:188-198;1986.
37. C.W. Pinson, A. Cobanoglu, M.T. Metzdorff, et al: Late surgical results for ischemic mitral regurgitation: Role of wall motion score and severity of regurgitation. *J Thorac Cardiovasc Surg* 88:663-672;1984.
38. N.W. Salomon, E.B. Stinson, R.B. Griepp, et al: Patient-related risk factors as predictors of results following isolated mitral valve replacement. *Ann Thorac Surg* 24:519-530;1977.

39. J.S. Chaffin, W.M. Daggett: Mitral valve replacement: A 9-year follow-up of risks and survivals. *Ann Thorac Surg* 27:312-319;1979.
40. B.W. Lytle, D.M. Cosgrove, C.C. Gill, et al: Mitral valve replacement with myocardial revascularization; early and late results for 300 patients, 1970-1983. *Circulation* 71:1179-90;1985.
41. L.S.C. Czer, R.J. Gray, M.A. DeRobertis, et al: Mitral valve replacement: Impact of coronary artery disease and determinants of prognosis after revascularization. *Circulation* 70:1198-1207;1984.
42. V.J. DiSesa, L.H. Cohn, J.J. Collins, et al: Determinants of operative survival following combined mitral valve replacement and coronary revascularization. *Ann Thorac Surg* 34:482-489;1982.
43. E. Rapaport: Natural history of aortic and mitral valve disease. *Am J Cardiol* 35:221-7;1979.
44. W.L. Proudfit, A.V.G. Bruschke, F.M. Sones, Jr.: Natural history of obstructive coronary artery disease: ten-year study of 601 nonsurgical cases. *Prog Cardiovasc Dis* 21:53-78;1978.
45. B.W. Lytle: Combined surgery for valve and coronary artery disease. *Clive Clin J Med* 55:79-87;1988.
46. J.A. Magovern, J.L. Pennock, D.B. Campbell, et al: Aortic valve replacement and combined aortic valve replacement and coronary artery bypass grafting: predicting high risk groups. *J Am Coll Cardiol* 9:38-43;1987.
47. J.K. Kirklin, D.C. Naftel, E.H. Blackstone, J.W. Kirklin, R.C. Brown: Risk factors for mortality after primary combined valvular and coronary artery surgery. *Circulation* 79:I185-90;1989.
48. B.W. Lytle, D.M. Cosgrove, C.C. Gill, et al: Aortic valve replacement combined with myocardial revascularization. Late results and determinants of risk for 471 in-hospital survivors. *J Thorac Cardiovasc Surg* 95:402-14;1988.

CARDIAC ANESTHESIA AND OXYGEN DELIVERY AND UPTAKE IN THE CRITICALLY ILL

T. James Gallagher M.D.

University of Florida College of Medicine
Shands Hospital
Gainesville, Florida

This chapter will include a discussion of anesthetic agents used in cardiac anesthesia, as well as a discussion on oxygen transport in the critically ill patient. Other specific aspects such as cardiopulmonary bypass will be found elsewhere.

CARDIAC ANESTHESIA

Induction Agents

Cardiac anesthesia, like all general anesthetics is often begun with the use of an induction agent to rapidly render the patient unconscious. These agents may be narcotics alone or in combination with benzodiazepines, short-acting anesthetics, or in some cases the agent selected to be used for maintenance of anesthesia during the case.

Thiopental

The most common agent used to induce anesthesia is sodium thiopental. Bolus administration of the agent results in high drug levels to the brain with the resulting unconsciousness and analgesia. The agent is relatively short-acting because of its rapid redistribution to the less well perfused tissues such as muscle and ultimately fat. Disappearance from the central blood volume as it is redistributed results in rapid dissipation of action. Significant enzyme induction

Cardiac Surgery: Current Issues, Edited by A.C. Cernaianu
and A.J. DelRossi Plenum Press, New York, 1992

occurs with chronic alcohol intake. These patients almost always require higher dosages to induce anesthesia. Sodium thiopental depresses cardiovascular function. It not only decreases cardiac contractility, but it also acts as a potent vasodilating agent. Both properties can contribute to a decrease in blood pressure and cardiac output.

Thiopental can depress respiratory function and will shift the CO_2 response curve to the right. Bronchospasm is often thought to be a complication following administration of thiopental. However, almost always, this problem develops secondary to light anesthesia, rather than any allergic reaction.

Etomidate

Etomidate is another single dose agent often used to induce anesthesia. The initial distribution half life is approximately three minutes with this agent. Most of its therapeutic effects appear to be dissipated within ten minutes of administration.

A major purported advantage of etomidate is its minimal effects upon cardiovascular function. Etomidate has minimal analgesic properties and therefore may not block the cardiovascular response to various interventions. Etomidate may depress the CO_2 response curve but not to the degree commonly seen with barbiturate agents. The agent is primarily cleared by the liver.

Propofol

Propofol is an alkylphenol with hypnotic properties. The agent is lipid soluble and is suspended in a fat emulsion which serves as a delivery vehicle. The initial distribution half life of propofol varies between two and eight minutes. Propofol will cause vasodilatation and can reduce blood pressure. As an induction dose it may have minimal analgesic properties and various procedures may result in a reflex hypertension.

Propofol will depress respiration in a manner similar to barbiturates. Apnea has been detected following an induction dose.

Benzodiazepines

Benzodiazepines such as midazolam have also been used to induce anesthesia. These are often combined with narcotics in that regard. Benzodiazepines can both depress blood pressure and cardiac contractility. This appears to be a dose related response and is more likely to occur in patients already debilitated. Cardiovascular depression is also more common when benzodiazepines are combined with narcotics.

Benzodiazepines can also produce apnea, particularly when combined with narcotic agents. In small dosages, they can induce anesthesia particularly in debilitated patients.

Maintenance of Anesthesia

After induction of anesthesia the anesthesiologist must maintain anesthesia for the duration of the operative procedure. This can usually be accomplished either with volatile anesthetic gases or narcotic agents. Often a combination of both are used in an attempt to minimize the detrimental effects of both groups.

Volatile Anesthetic Agents

Volatile inhalation agents provide a rapid onset and rapid dissipation of action. Drug uptake and drug excretion occur through the lungs and are a function of alveolar ventilation and cardiac output. Since this is a continuous administration, the drug can be titrated to the appropriate effect.

The major inhalation agents currently available include halothane, ethane, and forane. All three provide appropriate and desired levels of general anesthesia. Nitrous oxide is a fourth inhalation agent. While not capable by itself of providing general anesthesia, it can reduce the required dosage of the other inhalation agents and does provide some sleep effects with minimal analgesia.

The most common agent used in cardiovascular anesthesia is isoforane. Isoforane, like the other two halogenated agents, ethane and halothane, is a potent peripheral vasodilator and can depress cardiac function. Both responses appear to be dose related. Isoforane can produce a coronary steal type syndrome in a patient with underlying myocardial disease.

All inhalation agents depress respiratory function. While spontaneous respiration may be preserved both tidal volume and minute ventilation decrease. There also appears to be an alteration in the CO_2 response curve with a shift to the right.

The inhalation agents also interface with neuromuscular function and may result in some degree of peripheral muscular weakness, with a resultant decrease in required neuromuscular blockade requirements.

Nitrous oxide by itself appears to have minimal effects upon cardiac function. However, in the debilitated heart, particularly in combination with narcotics, it can depress contractility. In general, nitrous oxide has fallen in more disfavor among anesthesiologists, and its use appears to be continually decreasing.

The solubility of nitrous oxide promotes diffusion into air containing spaces. This may include microemboli within the vascular system. During cardiac surgery procedures this can contribute to an expansion of these bubbles and result in various degrees of vaso-occlusion.

Narcotics

The most common narcotics used during cardiac anesthesia include morphine, fentanyl, sufentanil, and alfentanil. Major advantages of narcotics include less depression of cardiac contractility. The products also appear to preserve autoregulation to heart and kidneys. They also can provide a degree of postoperative analgesia.

Potential disadvantages of narcotics include occasional hypotension seen on induction. Fentanyl in particular can induce muscle rigidity requiring muscle relaxants to enable the anesthesiologist to ventilate the patient. Narcotics may also prolong the recovery time resulting in prolonged mechanical ventilation in the postoperative period.

Narcotics can be used alone or in combination with nitrous oxide to provide anesthesia. They may also be used in combination with other inhalation agents. This can result in less cardiovascular depression because of the reduced dosage requirements of the inhalation agent. All four agents can produce hypotension. Morphine related hypotension appears to be mediated as much by histamine release as well as its direct effect upon sympathetic tone. Sufentanil and alfentanil appear to have direct action resulting in hypotension. All agents depress heart rate.

Respiratory depression is a common effect of all these agents. All shift the CO_2 response curve and hypoxic response curve to the right. In comparison to the other agents alfentanil and sufentanil appear to have the shortest duration of action.

OXYGEN DELIVERY AND UPTAKE IN THE CRITICALLY ILL

Clinicians often manipulate factors such as cardiac output in the critically ill. Ultimately we are interested in oxygen consumption and delivery. For each patient a delivery and oxygen consumption curve can be plotted. Initially this is a flow dependant relationship but beyond a certain critical oxygen. delivery there is no further increase in oxygen consumption (Figure 1). The shape and slope of the plot will vary depending upon the individual patient as well as the underlying metabolic status.

When delivery meets or exceeds oxygen demands the oxygen extraction remains in a predictable range (3.5-5.5 ml/dl). However delivery may decrease and fail to deliver sufficient oxygen to meet metabolic demands. This can occur because of a decrease in blood flow (cardiac output), a reduction in oxygen carrying capacity (hemoglobin), or a sudden increase in metabolic demands (shivering, hypothermia, etc.). Oxygen extraction will then utilize what we think of as the oxygen reserves. This will manifest itself as an increase in the oxygen extraction and widened arterial venous oxygen content difference $C(a\text{-}v)O_2$. Since cellular oxygen uptake remains diffusion dependant, a lower limit of venous oxygen content exists below which no further oxygen can be removed. When these reserves have been completely expended anaerobic metabolism and lactic acidosis result. The increase in oxygen extraction is the normal physiologic response to increased demands in the face of reduced delivery. The acidosis signifies the exhaustion of the available oxygen reserves.

The increased oxygen extraction manifested by an increased $C(a\text{-}v)O_2$ causes concern because it represents a global measurement. Unfortunately this information does not provide any specific data regarding any particular vascular bed such as a liver, kidney, brain or gut. Under normal conditions, organs such as the heart already demonstrate a maximum extraction of oxygen; therefore, the clinician should become concerned when global measurements reflect an overall increase in oxygen extraction. It is unclear what happens to organs such as the heart if there is an overall global increase in oxygen extraction. We can presume that the risk of ischemia significantly increases under such circumstances.

Patient situations in which the above scenario might develop include those unable to increase cardiac output and/or with reduced oxygen carrying capacity. This is often combined with increased metabolic demands such as develops with generalized sepsis, multiple organ failure, or following major operative procedures.

Specialized clinical circumstances such as general anesthesia result in an overall decrease in oxygen consumption and oxygen requirements. This helps explain why anesthetized patients do not develop such metabolic problems despite a decrease in cardiac output and often blood pressure.

Other clinical circumstances have been associated with a decrease in oxygen consumption and as a corollary a significant narrowing of the $C(a\text{-}v)O_2$. A small percentage of patients with generalized sepsis particularly in the late stages may demonstrate a cellular inability to extract and utilize oxygen. The cellular respiration appears "paralyzed". This predicts a bad outcome and generally has an associated metabolic acidosis.

Peripheral shunting such as with an arterial venous fistula will also result in an increased venosus oxygen content and narrowed $C(a\text{-}v)O_2$ difference. This may be seen as in a traumatic arterial venous fistula following injury to the femoral vessels. Another clinical example might be a patient with hepatic cirrhosis and arterial venous shunting throughout the liver. Cyanide toxicity can develop after large dose or long term of sodium nitroprusside administration. The cyanide inactivates the cytochrome P-450 system. Again cellular respiration is arrested and venous oxygen content significantly increases. Lactic acidosis often accompanies this situation. Carbon monoxide acts in a similar fashion.

Current controversies in the care of the critically ill patient with sepsis or multiple system trauma, or following major operative procedures concern the degree to which oxygen consumption and delivery should be maximized. As previously stated, the metabolic requirements in this group of patients are higher. Delivery can often be driven to greater levels before the uncoupling of flow dependent oxygen consumption begins. Some clinicians cite recent literature which might suggest that early maximization of oxygen consumption by increased oxygen delivery will result in improved outcome. Shoemaker and colleagues have published data to suggest that in the early stages of resuscitation an oxygen deficit exists.[1] Survival and the degree of organ failure and complications appear related to the rapidity in which the oxygen debt can be eliminated. Patient demise is associated with failure to reverse this trend.

One interpretation would presume that the delay in resuscitation results in increased organ failure. On the other hand, preexisting or early development of organ failure, although not yet clinically recognized may preclude the clinicians' ability to reverse the situation as rapidly as in those patients who do not develop any organ failure. Initial resuscitation data in other studies demonstrates a clear delineation between survivors and nonsurvivors when both oxygen consumption and oxygen delivery are plotted. Shoemaker, et al. have further demonstrated a linear relationship of oxygen consumption measured early in the patient's course and plotted against survival.[2]

However, problems exist with these data. There are no control groups. The degree of resuscitation did vary on a patient to patient basis and the underlying diseases were not well controlled for. Furthermore, it is unclear that data gathered in the initial hours of the patient's arrival in the intensive care unit can be correlated that closely to outcome following a long term stay in the ICU.

Later data by this same group suggests that oxygen consumption had little if any relation to prediction of outcome.[3] While oxygen consumption was identical in both survivors and nonsurvivors, there was a slight decrease in delivery to nonsurvivors. This resulted in a slight increase in oxygen extraction. This data contrasts with the previous data, where outcome related much more closely to oxygen consumption.

Tuchschmidt studied patients admitted to a medical intensive care unit with a diagnosis of septic shock.[4] Plots of oxygen consumption against oxygen delivery failed to show a strong correlation between maximization of oxygen delivery, consumption and outcome. Above a certain critical oxygen delivery all patients survived, overall this represented a small percentage of patients. Below this level there were equal numbers of survivors and deaths. One can presume that there is no clear cut relationship between delivery, oxygen consumption and outcome.

Bakker's group in Europe also looked at patients with multiple system failure and plotted cardiac index, oxygen delivery, oxygen consumption and lactate.[5] Data were collected upon ICU admission and at the time of death or the last measurement prior to removal of the pulmonary artery catheter. There were no differences in the initial values for survivors and nonsurvivors, Furthermore, the final measurements at the time of maximum improvement or just prior to death again demonstrated no statistically significant difference in any of these parameters. However, nonsurvivors initially had a higher lactate level and were unable to clear it during the resuscitation period. This data may reflect a decrease in overall metabolic demands as patients improved versus a continued increase in those patients who died. The continued acidosis in the nonsurvivors may represent cellular failure. Oxygen consumption and delivery remained identical at all times in both groups.

The conflicts in this and other data,[6-8] presently make it difficult to promote or support one mode of therapy. In my opinion, the lack of clear cut relationship of maximization of oxygen consumption and delivery to outcome precludes attempts to perform these manipulations in each and every patient at risk. This is particularly so in the elderly, since many may have underlying coronary artery disease.

A clinician can only minimally influence oxygen carrying capacity. Therefore, most maneuvers are designed to increase cardiac output. Often the elderly heart cannot respond or actually may be compromised and develop increased oxygen demands in excess of the increase of available delivery. Oxygen delivery can be increased as necessary to maximal levels by several different manipulations. These include increased oxygen carrying capacity (hemoglobin), shifts of the oxyhemoglobin dissociation curve (Bohr effect) and manipulation of cardiac output. A simple increase in hemoglobin can significantly improve oxygen delivery.[9] In terms of physiologic cost, this represents a much cheaper modality than manipulations to increase cardiac output. For the acutely ill patient with multisystem failure I recommend a hemoglobin level of 11 to 13 gm/dl. At normothermia this will not impact on viscosity or compromise microcirculatory flow. However, it does minimize cardiac work requirements. Furthermore, blood acts as an excellent intervascular volume expander.

Little manipulation of the oxyhemoglobin dissociation curve be clinically achieved. However, a rightward shift in the face of mild acidosis will enhance oxygen extraction. Alkalosis has between associated with an increase in both cardiac arrhythmias and work of breathing and other problems.

Maneuvers to enhance cardiac output must be weighed against potential increases in myocardial oxygen consumption sometimes to detrimental effects. In general, enhancement of cardiac filling pressures or preload usually has minimal effect on increased oxygen consumption. Utilizing the standard monitoring devices the clinician would construct a cardiac function curve based on filling or wedge pressures. Normally, maximal cardiac output will occur at wedge pressures of between 15-18 mmHg.

Cardiac work against an elevated impedance such as manifested by an increased systemic vascular resistance will increase myocardial wall tension and hence afterload. However, the physician should recognize that systemic vascular resistance represents a calculated rather than a measured value. It will always vary inversely to cardiac output. As such, cardiac output significantly influences this value.

We do not ordinarily measure cardiac contractility. Rather we infer depressed contractility when afterload and preload have been optimized yet cardiac output still appears to be inadequate. This situation would usually warrant the use of an inotropic agent. However, on occasion this may be associated with an increase in oxygen consumption and potential myocardial ischemia.

While rate can sometimes increase cardiac output in the elderly, debilitated patient, it will often cause significant myocardial ischemia. For that reason, heart rates of 100 or less per minute should remain the target. Higher rates have an increased incidence of myocardial ischemia, particularly in patients with underlying coronary artery disease.

In summary, the clinician should primarily concern his or her effort in the critically ill patient with optimization of oxygen consumption by appropriate enhancement of oxygen delivery. It is unclear whether or not maximization of oxygen consumption can ultimately result in any improvement in survival. It seems best at this time to recommend adequate oxygen consumptions as represented by normal arterial venous content and the lack of lactic acidosis. This should be accomplished at the least expense to myocardial function.

REFERENCES

1. R.D. Bland, W.C. Shoemaker, E. Abraham, et a: Hemodynamic and oxygen transport patterns in surviving and nonsurviving patients. *Crit Care Med* 13:85-90;1985.
2. R.D. Bland, W.C. Shoemaker: Common physiologic patterns in general surgical patients. *Surgical Clinics of North America,* 65 793-809;1985.
3. W.C. Shoemaker, P.L. Appel, H.B. Kram, et al: Prospective trial of supranormal values of survivors as therapeutic goals in high risk surgical patients. *Chest* 94:1176-86;1988.
4. J. Tuchschmidt, D. Oblitas, J.C. Fried: Oxygen consumption in Sepsis and Septic Shock. *Crit Care Med* 19:664-671;1991.
5. J. Bakker, M. Coffernils, M. Leon, et al: Blood lactate levels are superior to oxygen derived values in predicting outcome in human septic shock. *Chest* 99:956-62;1991.
6. W.C. Shoemaker, P.L. Appel, H.B. Kram: Incidence, physiologic description, compensatory mechanisms, and therapeutic implications of monitored events. *Crit Care Med* 17:1277-85;1989.
7. J.A. Kruse, M.T. Haupt, V.K. Puri, et al: Lactate levels as predictors of the relationship between oxygen delivery and consumption in ARDS. *Chest* 98:959-962;1990.
8. J. Pakker, J.L. Vincent: The oxygen supply dependency phenomenon is associated with increased blood lactate levels. *J Critical Care* 6:15259;1991.
9. C.P. Steffes, J.S. Bender, M.A. Levison: Blood transfusion in oxygen consumption in surgical sepsis. *Crit Care Med* 19:512-17;1991.

COMPLEX CARDIAC SURGERY

Denton A. Cooley, M.D.

Texas Heart Institute
University of Texas Medical School
Houston, Texas

During the past several decades, impressive progress has been made in cardiovascular surgery. Correction of most lesions and anomalies has become routine. Some of the more complex problems, however, still challenge the surgeon. In some instances, procedures that were once routine, such as coronary artery bypass, have become more complex. In the case of coronary bypass, this change occurred as surgeons began to search for better bypass conduits. This report describes a few of these complex problems.

CORONARY ARTERY DISEASE

Two major developments caused an explosion of heart surgery: simplification of cardiopulmonary bypass and selective coronary arteriography. Because of limited knowledge of coronary anatomy, surgical treatment for coronary artery disease did not become practical until 1958, when Mason Sones[1] introduced selective coronary arteriography, which became the key to direct revascularization of the ischemic myocardium. Four years earlier, surgical treatment of coronary artery disease had become a possibility, when John Gibbon[2] operated on a patient by using cardiopulmonary bypass. Unfortunately, the earliest operations had to be performed with an elaborate extracorporeal system and large volumes of homologous blood for priming. In 1962, however, we[3] published our initial report describing a simplified technique of cardiopulmonary bypass that used disposable plastic oxygenators, 5% dextrose prime, and normothermia. An explosive increase in the volume of cardiac surgery ensued, fueled mainly by the coronary artery bypass procedure.

The pioneers of coronary artery bypass surgery included names

Cardiac Surgery: Current Issues, Edited by A.C. Cernaianu and A.J. DelRossi Plenum Press, New York, 1992

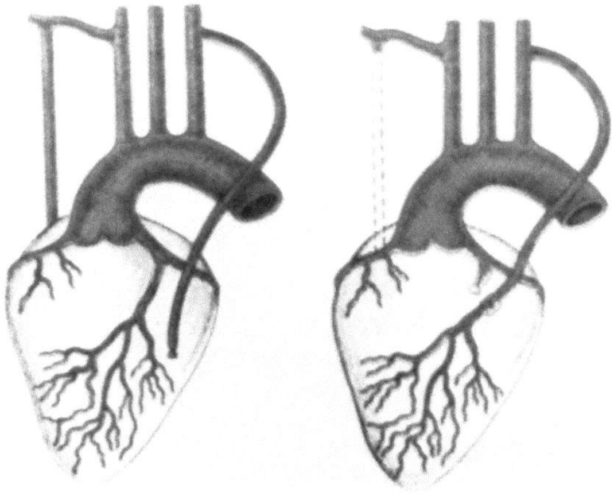

Figure 1. Suture anastomosis of the internal mammary artery (Demikhov).

such as Bailey, Hallman and Cooley, Garrett, Sabiston, Favaloro, and Johnson. These last two pioneers probably did the most to convince members of the medical and surgical professions that coronary bypass was realistic. Through the work of all of these pioneers, we learned that coronary artery bypass could relieve symptoms such as angina and dysrhythmia, and could even prolong life expectancy.

Most of these initial operations were done with multiple saphenous vein grafts. Although the autologous saphenous vein has been used successfully for the bypass procedure, these veins are often subject to premature degenerative and sclerotic change, especially when they are subjected to arterial pressure. In a recently published study, ischemic symptoms returned in most patients within 15 to 20 years after coronary artery bypass grafting.[4] However, this recurrence of symptoms was most likely to manifest as a return of angina and, only rarely, as sudden death. As a result of the problems associated with the saphenous vein, alternative conduits are now routinely used in conjunction

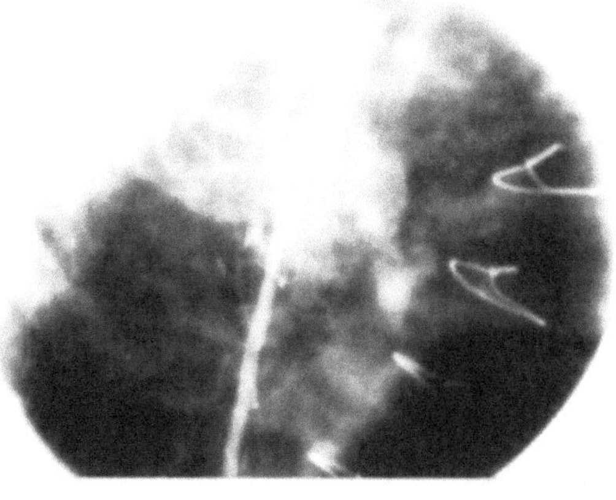

Figure 2. Angiogram showing patent left internal mammary artery bypass in a patient 5 years after surgery.

with or in place of the saphenous vein graft. Most often chosen is the internal mammary artery.

In 1952, Demikhov[5] in Russia conducted experiments in 15 dogs in which the internal mammary artery was sutured directly to the coronary artery below the site of a coronary artery lesion (Fig. 1). Demikhov's remarkable work showed that the internal mammary artery graft could remain patent in dogs for more than 3 years. In 1964, Vasilii Kolesov[6] of Leningrad performed the first sutured internal mammary-coronary artery anastomosis in a 44-year-old man with class III angina. Other investigators followed. Not until recently, however, has the internal mammary artery been used routinely in coronary artery bypass operations (Fig. 2).

Based on the success of the internal mammary artery, surgeons have continued to look for other suitable arterial conduits and, as a result, the right gastroepiploic (Fig. 3) and inferior epigastric arteries are now being more widely used for coronary artery bypass operations.

At the Texas Heart Institute, we have already performed more than 50,000 coronary bypass operations (Table 1). These operations, however, are not without risk. Currently recognized risk factors include urgency of surgery, age of the patient, and previous cardiac operations. However, factors such as female sex, left ventricular ejection fraction, and left main coronary disease are not considered as great a risk as they were even 5 years ago.

In the last 10 years, the characteristics of our patient population have changed. For example, in 1977, 14% of our patients were women, 32% were more than 60 years old, 5.5% were more than 70 years old, and only 2.9% had undergone a previous coronary artery bypass operation. In contrast, in 1987, 19% of our patients were women, 53%

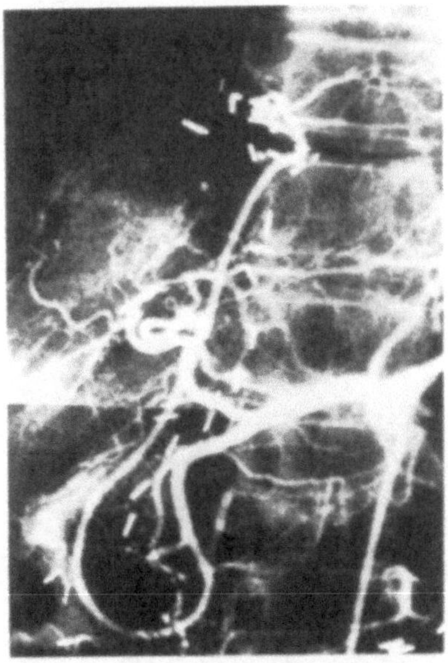

Figure 3. Coronary bypass using the gastroepiploic artery as a conduit.

TABLE 1. Surgical Procedures, Texas Heart Institute, 1975-1990.

Number of Procedures Performed	
Surgical	
Cardiac	
Coronary artery bypass	50,003
Other coronary	1,330
Cardiac transplantation	415
Congenital	13,169
Valvular	16,078
Other cardiac	34,175
Total Cardiac	115,170
Vascular, non-cardiac	25,783
Non-cardiovascular	16,562
Total Surgical	157,515
Percutaneous transluminal coronary angioplasty (PTCA)	8,756
Cardiac Catheterization	119,324

TABLE 2. Surgical Procedures, Texas Heart Institute, 1990.

Number of Procedures Performed	
Surgical	
Cardiac	
Coronary artery bypass	2,456
Other coronary	118
Cardiac transplantation	47
Congenital	779
Valvular	743
Other cardiac	3,055
Total Cardiac	7,198
Vascular, non-cardiac	1,737
Non-cardiovascular	1,449
Total Surgical	10,384
Percutaneous transluminal coronary angioplasty (PTCA)	1,315
Cardiac Catheterization	8,984

were more then 60 years old, and 18% were more than 70 years old. By 1987, 15.9% had undergone a previous coronary artery bypass operation, an increase of 13%. Thus, because our patient population is becoming older and sicker, the overall operative risk has increased rather than decreased, as would be expected with increasing experience.

The face of coronary artery bypass was significantly changed in 1974, when Andreas Gruentzig[7] introduced percutaneous transluminal coronary angioplasty (PTCA) to treat coronary stenosis, primarily for patients with single-vessel disease. With increasing sophistication of equipment and experience of operators, indications for PTCA have expanded to patients with multivessel disease and more complex lesions. Primary success rates are reported at 90% to 95%, but, unfortunately, restenosis occurs in 30% to 35% of patients within 6 months.[8,9] In addition, complications occur in approximately 10% of patients. Nevertheless, when the final numbers are reported for 1990, the growth in angioplasty in the United States is anticipated to have reached 300,000 procedures. Between 1975 and 1991, cardiologists at the Texas Heart Institute performed 8,756 PTCA procedures. In 1990, cardiologists performed 1,315 PTCA procedures, while surgeons performed 2,456 coronary artery bypass procedures. Although the number

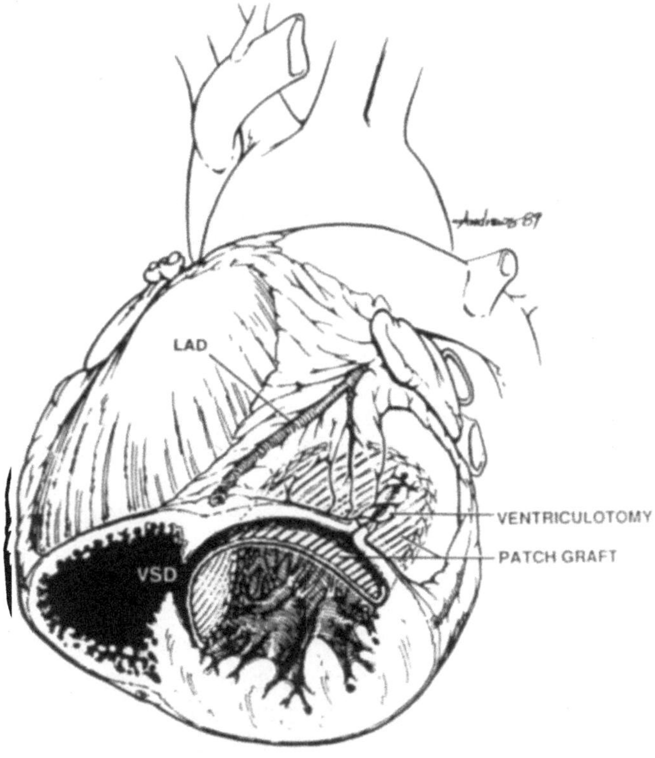

Figure 4. Internal placement of a Dacron fabric graft covering the infarcted myocardium. The patch in this instance covers a septal perforation (LAD = left anterior descending coronary artery; VSD = ventricular septal defect). Reprinted with permission of the Annals of Thoracic Surgery 1990;49:150.

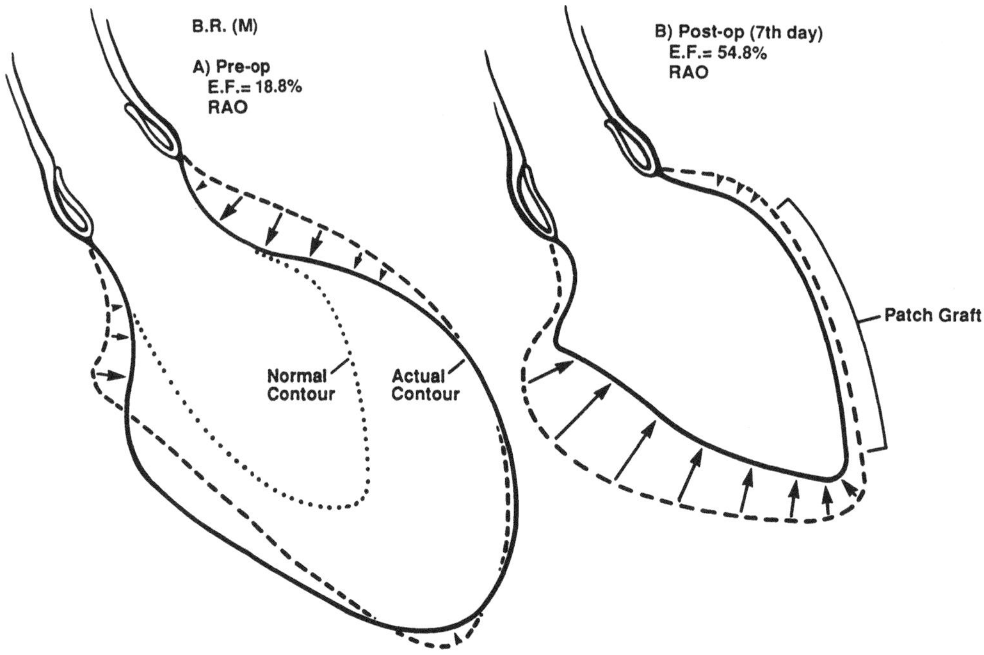

Figure 5. Preoperative and postoperative angiographic representations showing a 36% increase in ejection fraction in a patient 7 days following left ventricular endoaneurysmorrhaphy.

of patients treated with coronary artery bypass has decreased, the total number of patients undergoing direct treatment of coronary lesions has remained about the same.

Even though PTCA has resulted in fewer patients being treated by coronary artery bypass, the bypass procedure remains the definitive treatment for patients with severe atherosclerotic lesions. Although palliative, coronary artery bypass effectively relieves angina, increases exercise capacity, and prolongs life in certain subsets of patients, including those patients with left main coronary disease, 3-vessel coronary disease, 2-vessel coronary disease with a proximal occlusion of the left anterior descending coronary artery, and high-risk subsets with resting or stress-induced ischemia. Therefore, bypass surgery is best reserved for those at increased risk.

COMPLICATIONS OF CORONARY OCCLUSION

Treating the complications of acute myocardial infarction continues to challenge surgeons. One such complication is ventricular aneurysm. As with coronary artery bypass, surgical treatment of these lesions became feasible after the introduction of cardiopulmonary bypass. In 1958, we performed the first excision of a left ventricular aneurysm.[10] After that procedure, we repaired approximately 2,500 ventricular aneurysms by using cardiopulmonary bypass and a number of modifi-

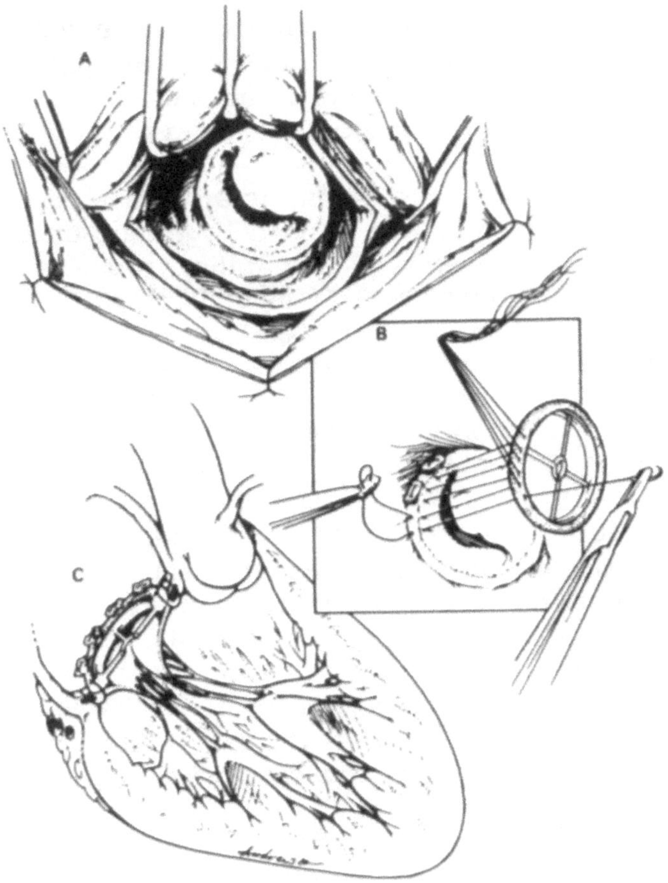

Figure 6. Intravalvular implantation of a low-profile mechanical prosthesis in the mitral position (see text).

cations of the original technique, ending with a linear repair and excision.

In recent years, we have modified and improved repair of ventricular aneurysms by using intracavitary endoaneurysmorrhaphy.[11,12] This technique, which is similar to that reported by Dor[13] and Jatene,[14] makes the repair more anatomic. We use an oval patch of Dacron fabric or bovine pericardium. As a result, the suture line restores shape, contour, and volume to the left ventricle (Fig. 4). The patch used in the repair compartmentalizes the left ventricle, potentially creating an additional intracavitary space. This space is incorporated into the ventricular wall, which probably accounts for the good functional result seen on follow up of the patients (Fig. 5). Maintaining the surface anatomy permits normal left ventricular function, eliminates paradoxical contractile forces, and facilitates coronary bypass. While the noncontractile patch admittedly plays a purely passive role, it serves to stabilize ventricular contraction during systole. The technique of endoaneurysmorrhaphy can be extended to areas of localized myocardial fibrosis not necessarily identified as an aneurysm, but with reduced left ventricular function. The concept can also be applied to calcified aneurysms and to aneurysms on the posterior ventricular surface, since the clinical and functional results with this method have been improved.

Another complication of myocardial infarction is mitral regurgitation. Mitral regurgitation can be caused by dilatation of the mitral annulus, by triggering ischemia of the papillary muscles that produce irregular closure of the mitral leaflets, or by forcing a frank rupture of a papillary muscle or chordae tendineae. Whenever possible, we repair rather than replace the mitral valve in instances of regurgitation.

Valvuloplasty can be performed several ways. We most commonly use a valvuloplasty ring, although we still occasionally perform commissural plication. The objective of both methods is to reduce the circumference of the mitral annulus. If a partial rupture of the posterior leaflet has occurred, the flail scallop is excised, the remaining leaflet is repaired, and the annulus is reduced and supported by a circumferential fabric ring. When the anterior leaflet interferes with flow, the leaflet can be incised and tacked back to the side of the annulus. This procedure keeps the papillary muscle intact, giving it needed support. When mitral regurgitation is associated with ventricular aneurysm, we use endoaneurysmorrhaphy to relieve the dysfunction. By restoring the normal position of the papillary muscles, mitral dysfunction can be relieved.

When replacement is necessary, we use a technique of intravalvular implantation of a low-profile mechanical prosthesis (Fig 6).[15] This technique preserves the anterior and posterior chordae and papillary mechanisms, which may decrease the incidence of postoperative left ventricular dysfunction that has been noted following standard mitral valve replacement.[16-18] Today, much experience has been gained with both mechanical and bioprosthetic valves. For both types of valves, there are advantages and disadvantages. Bioprostheses are not as durable as mechanical valves and are associated with more complications, especially calcification. We now prefer mechanical valves in most situations.[19] Many designs are made with pyrolytic carbon, which has proved to be a very durable material. These new valves have wider openings, and, thus, there is minimal regurgitation. The only disadvantage of these new mechanical valves continues to be the need for anticoagulation to prevent thromboembolism.

AORTIC ANEURYSMS

Aortic aneurysms have long challenged cardiovascular surgeons. The first direct attack on these lesions came in the early 1950s, when we[20] excised a sacciform aneurysm of the thoracic aorta and arch by using tangential excision with lateral aortorrhaphy. Tangential excision and lateral repair were satisfactory techniques for sacciform lesions when less than 50% of the aortic circumference was involved by the aneurysm. Fusiform lesions, however, proved more difficult, since vascular grafts were in limited supply and were mostly fresh or preserved homografts. With the evolution of fabric grafts made of synthetic fibers, excision with graft replacement became standard.

The method we currently use to repair aortic aneurysms disregards excision of the aneurysmal wall and instead employs the objective of relining the aneurysm with a sturdy fabric graft preclotted with autologous plasma.[21] After the aorta is rendered bloodless by circulatory arrest during induced hypothermia to levels of 22-24° C, the internal reconstruction is performed with a fabric graft. By using open repair distally, total circulatory arrest can usually be limited to less than 20 minutes. Once the distal anastomosis has been accomplished, a clamp is placed on the woven Dacron tube, and circulation is restored from the femoral arterial cannulation. The proximal anastomosis is then done at the appropriate level, while body temperature is restored to normal. Thus, pulsatile circulation is restored to the patient's entire body. By leaving the wall of the aneurysm intact, anatomic structures such as the lung, phrenic and vagus nerves, duodenum and left kidney are not disturbed, and the limited dissection reduces blood loss.

Considerations in treatment of aneurysms of the ascending aorta involve the assessment of the proximal and distal extent of the lesion and of the involvement of the aortic valve. Atherosclerosis is a major cause of aneurysms in this location. Aneurysms resulting from a defect in the elastic tissues known as Erdheim's cystic medionecrosis are, however, increasing in frequency. Aneurysms resulting from medial degeneration are generally located at the base of the heart, involve the proximal ascending aorta, and, frequently, include coronary sinuses to varying degrees. The annulus and aortic valve leaflets are also often involved in the disease process. Most aneurysms that result from medial degeneration are fusiform. These aneurysms are susceptible to a number of serious complications, most notably rupture and aortic valvular insufficiency, and need to be treated on an urgent basis.

For acute dissecting ascending aortic aneurysms, the same techniques can be applied. In most cases, the adventitial and intimal layers can be sutured together, thereby obliterating the false lumen. Reinforcement of the distal suture line with an external wrap by using a Dacron vascular graft or felt strip is advisable. Other centers have used a ringed intraluminal graft[22,23] to treat dissecting aneurysms. The intraluminal graft is inserted into the true lumen of the dissected aorta, and the aorta is circumferentially ligated against the groove in the rings.

Even with aneurysms of the transverse arch, we use moderate levels of hypothermia and a brief period of circulatory arrest, although upon reaching these levels of hypothermia, usually the patient's temperature further declines to 18-20° C. In our patients, deep hypothermia has been associated with problems.[24] Prolonged periods of cardiopulmonary bypass are needed for the cooling and rewarming phases of deep hypothermia. Prolonged bypass and hypothermia interfere with normal coagulation mechanisms and may produce troublesome bleeding in some patients. We have also seen multiple organ system dysfunction postoperatively after a technically satisfactory operation, which raises doubts regarding the level of protection afforded by this technique.

When the lesion involves only the proximal portion of the transverse arch, a long, oblique anastomosis is done when necessary to restore continuity to the brachiocephalic arteries and the descending thoracic aorta. If, however, the lesion extends into the distal portion of the transverse arch, the distal anastomosis is done separately, and the brachiocephalic arteries are implanted as a large patch into the convexity of the graft (Fig. 7). Once the distal anastomoses have been completed, the clamp is placed on the graft. After blood fills the aorta and the brachiocephalic vessels, air is eliminated. Most such repairs can be accomplished within a period of 30 minutes of circulatory arrest.[25] The proximal anastomosis into the ascending aorta may then be undertaken with less urgency or haste.

CONDUCTION SYSTEM

Pacemakers

Since cardiac pacemakers were clinically introduced in 1963,[26] improvements in technology have caused remarkable changes in the available therapy. The initial indications were only for patients with bradycardia and resultant syncope, but the clinician now has a wide choice of pacemakers and, thus, an increased number of conditions in

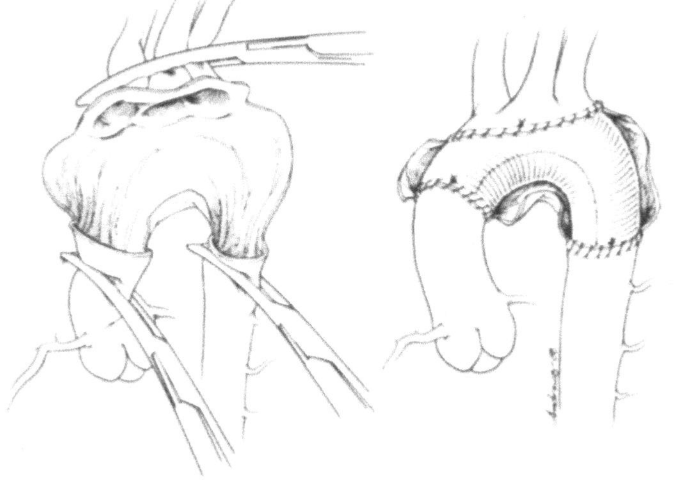

Figure 7. Repair of an aneurysm of the transverse aortic arch.

which their use may be beneficial. The technologic advances have included multiprogrammable single and dual-chambered pacemakers, long-lived atrial and ventricular leads, and activity-sensing, rate-modulated and temperature-based, rate-responsive pacing. Programmability and memory are now telemetry-based.

The development of physiological pacemakers has occurred simultaneously with several other trends in cardiac pacing. Presently, available pacemakers are smaller and lighter than the devices of only a year or two ago. Devices are now physiologically contoured. Despite recently renewed interest in nuclear-powered pulse generators, modern pacing technology is nearly exclusively powered by batteries of lithium chemistry, a situation not likely to change soon.

Tachyarrhythmias

Definitive and curative surgical procedures are currently available for most of the important types of tachyarrhythmias. In children, these techniques have evolved over the relatively brief period of 15-20 years to a state where precise electrophysiologic diagnosis is possible, and the surgical result is predictable and relatively safe.[27] The most significant recent advances have been accomplished in the area of computerized multiplex mapping, which allows rapid and precise calculation of conduction intervals at multiple points on the cardiac surface with data captured and stored during one cardiac cycle. Both palliative and curative operations have been developed and should be considered as therapy for children who are not thought to be at risk for sudden death, but whose lifestyles are severely altered as a result of their arrhythmias.

Wolff-Parkinson-White (WPW) syndrome, which causes supraventricular tachycardia, results from a direct atrioventricular muscle connection. Accessory A-V muscle bundles have been found on the right and left free walls as well as in the septum. The pathways are small, usually 10 mm in length and 1 mm in diameter.

Patients in whom WPW is suspected should undergo electrophysiologic study. The data obtained will direct the surgeon to one of four possible procedures: a left posterior dissection through the left atrium, a right anterolateral dissection through the right atrium, a posterior septal dissection and/or cryoablation, or, rarely, an anteroseptal dissection and cryoablation. The most common operation is the left posterior dissection.

Surgery is indicated in patients with a combination of syncope or cardiac arrest, atrial fibrillation, and a short refractory period of the Kent bundle. We generally attempt to defer operation until after 2 years of age, since SVT may disappear and catheter mapping, especially entering the coronary sinus, is more difficult at this age. Nevertheless, we have performed successful surgery in an infant as young as 3 months.

Tricuspid Atresia

In his original report of a new technique for correction of tricuspid atresia, Fontan[29] described insertion of a valved conduit to achieve continuity between the right atrium and pulmonary artery. A second valve was placed in the inferior vena cava (IVC) to prevent reflux blood into the IVC during atrial systole. Problems associated with valves and conduits, however, led others to develop successful modifications of the original procedure.[30-32] Some patients have a left superior vena cava (LSVC) draining either into the coronary sinus or the left atrium. Suggested techniques to deal with this entity include ligation of the LSVC, construction of a left-sided Glenn shunt, or more complicated intra-atrial baffles to redirect blood flow from the LSVC into the right atrium.[33,34]

de Leval and associates[35] modified Fontan's procedure by excluding most or all of the right atrium from the systemic venous return. The potential advantages of this technique included simplicity and easy reproducibility, avoidance of injury to the atrioventricular node, and prevention of right atrial distension, thereby reducing the possibility of early and late arrhythmias and atrial thrombosis. We have further modified this concept by utilizing the LSVC as a drainage channel to direct blood from the IVC to the pulmonary arteries.[36] We place a glutaraldehyde-treated autogenous pericardial baffle or a suitable prosthetic patch baffle to direct blood flow from the IVC to the dilated coronary sinus. The operation is performed by using cardiopulmonary bypass with hypothermia and low flow or total circulatory arrest, depending on the age of the patient and the complexity of the condition. The baffle is sutured around the orifice of the IVC and anastomosed to the coronary sinus. The sutures are placed inside the anterior lip of the coronary sinus, thereby preventing injury to the atrioventricular node. The short length of the baffle lessens the risk of pulmonary venous obstruction, which can occur with other more complicated baffle techniques. The atrial septal defect is also enlarged if necessary.

Transposition of the Great Vessels

The development of two effective operations for correction of transposition of the great vessels was first reported by Senning[37] and later by Mustard,[38,39] both of whom described intracardiac repair of transposition of the great vessels. In both the Mustard and Senning procedures, the venous inflow into the ventricles is transposed by atrial inversion so that the left ventricle receives unoxygenated systemic venous blood, which is then pumped into the pulmonary artery. The right atrium and ventricle receive oxygenated pulmonary venous blood, which is then delivered into the ascending aorta. The actual surgical techniques differ considerably, but in concept the operations are the same. Since their introduction, numerous modifications of the original technique have been made by other contributors.

We prefer a modification of the Senning procedure, which has the advantage of avoiding biologic and synthetic patches. The operation can be performed expeditiously without patch augmentation of the septum.[40] In this procedure, the interatrial groove is opened in front of the right pulmonary veins and the left atrium is opened parallel to the right atrial incision. The atrial septum is fashioned into a flap by a U-shaped incision and the coronary sinus is cut back into the left atrium. When there is a large atrial septal defect or when balloon septostomy has been performed, the remaining atrial septal flap is unfolded by first making an endothelial incision at the base of the septal remnant on the left atrial side. This septal remnant is then unfolded to create a flap that is of adequate size to reach the required point anterior to the left pulmonary veins where they join the left atrium. This new septal flap is then sutured with running polypropylene suture between the

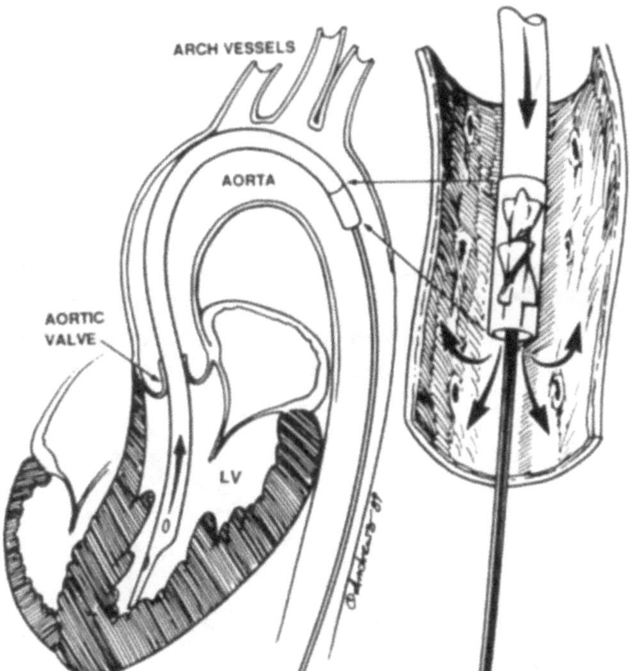

Figure 8. Position of the Hemopump in the left ventricle and aortic arch (LV, left ventricle). The Hemopump, which is the size of a pencil eraser, consists of a silicone inflow cannula, which is placed across the aortic valve, its tip being positioned in the left ventricle and its other end in the aorta. The aortic end encases a rotating screw that revolves up to 25,000 times per minute, thereby drawing blood from the left ventricle into the aorta and producing flows of up to 4.1 L/min. Reprinted with permission of the Annals of Thoracic Surgery 1989;48:733.

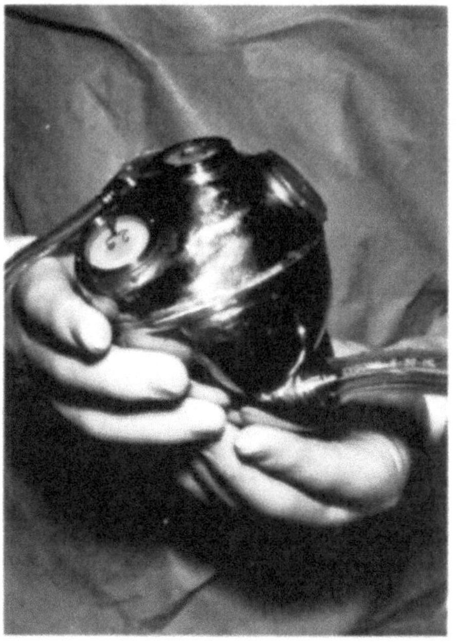

Figure 9. The Lapeyre artificial heart.

left pulmonary veins and the mitral valve, as usual.

Transposition can also be corrected by ventricular switch, using either the Jatene or Rastelli procedures. With the Jatene[41] technique, the pulmonary artery and aorta are interchanged, thus reversing the arterial outflow of the heart and creating an "anatomical" repair of the anomaly. This procedure has the theoretical advantage of at least maintaining the left ventricle as the systemic ventricle and the right ventricle as the normal pulmonary ventricle. The original technique described by Jatene usually involved use of a segment of fabric tube

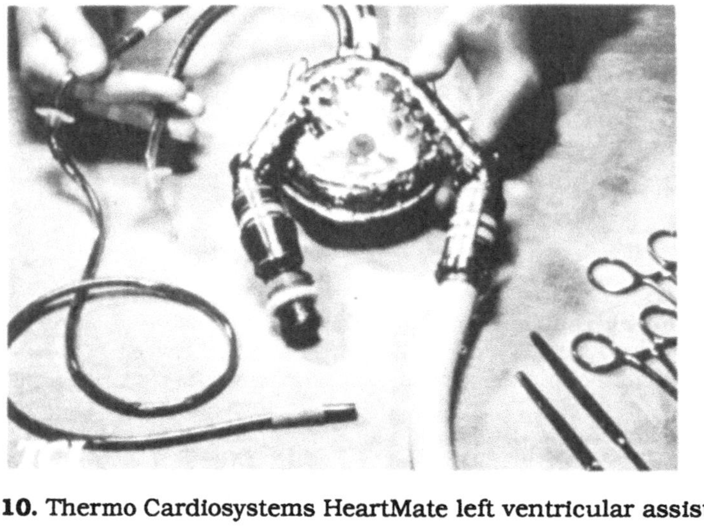

Figure 10. Thermo Cardiosystems HeartMate left ventricular assist device.

conduit to reestablish the continuity between the right ventricle and pulmonary artery. Lecompte[42] modified the approach, eliminating the need for the conduit. The main risk associated with the Jatene operation is the possibility of tension being placed on the coronary arteries. Another problem is that of establishing the left ventricle as the systemic ventricle if the left ventricle has only provided output to a low-pressure pulmonary arterial network. The Jatene procedure is mostly done in infants less than 6 weeks of age.

For patients with large ventricular septal defects and both pulmonary infundibular and valvular stenosis, the Rastelli[43] procedure is preferred. In this operation, the intracardiac ventricular septal repair is done to direct blood from the left ventricle through the large ventricular septal defect into the aortic valve and ascending aorta. A large Dacron patch is applied to form the tunnel or baffle to make this switch. In those patients with pulmonary valve atresia or severe infundibular stenosis, the proximal main pulmonary artery is ligated or the valve is oversewn. Once the ventricular passage has been completed, the outflow from the right ventricle to the pulmonary artery is completed with a fabric conduit. If the patient has increased pulmonary vascular resistance, then the outflow conduit should incorporate a valve.

TRANSPLANTATION AND MECHANICAL CIRCULATORY SUPPORT DEVICES

In the last decade, cardiac transplantation has gained wide acceptance as a definitive treatment for end-stage heart disease, with many centers reporting survival rates greater than 80% at 1 year. Since the introduction of cyclosporine to our transplant program in 1982, we have performed heart transplant operations in approximately 450 patients. After the introduction of cyclosporine, the number of transplant operations performed in adults increased immediately. In contrast, the number of pediatric heart transplantations increased slowly, primarily because most clinicians believed that such procedures, if performed at all, should be limited to older children. In 1984, however, surgeons at the Texas Heart Institute performed a heart transplant on an 8-month-old female infant with subendocardial fibroelastosis.[44] This little girl is now 7 years old, and despite immunosuppressive therapy, which included corticosteroids, she has continued to grow and develop normally.

The treatment of end-stage pediatric heart disease with heart transplantation has become routinely available only in the last several years. Between 1980 and 1988, 206 patients under 10 years of age had heart transplant operations compared with approximately 9000 patients over age 10 years.[45] In this group of young patients, the 30-day mortality rate was 25%. At Loma Linda University, Bailey has performed more than 60 transplants on babies with potentially fatal heart defects, many with univentricular heart. Survival rates for this more recent group have been comparable with those of adults. Rejection in these infant patients has been controlled with minimal doses of immunosuppressive agents.

The critical shortage of donor hearts, however, has meant that only 10% of patients who could benefit from the procedure are receiving transplants. In some patients, a long wait for a donor heart can result in profound end-organ dysfunction, which can jeopardize their status as transplant candidates. At the Texas Heart Institute, we have investigated several circulatory support devices to determine their effectiveness in supporting transplant candidates until a donor heart becomes available. The devices include the intra-aortic balloon pump (Datascope; Paramus, New Jersey), an extracorporeal centrifugal blood pump (BP-80, Bio-Medicus; Minneapolis, Minnesota), and the Hemopump (Fig. 8) (Nimbus; Rancho Cordova, California).

We have also successfully used the total artificial heart in staged transplant operations. In 1969, we first implanted a total artificial heart as a bridge to transplantation.[46] The TAH sustained the patient for 64 hours while we made a concerted effort to obtain an allograft for transplantation. The patient survived for 32 hours following transplantation before dying from infection. In 1981, the total artificial heart was used again for staged cardiac transplantation.[47] This second orthotopic implantation used an Akutsu-III TAH. The TAH pumped for 54 hours before an acceptable donor was found and we proceeded with cardiac transplantation. The patient lived for 7 1/2 days before dying from infection. Although the duration of life in these patients may not have been impressive, the experience indicated the clinical feasibility of total circulatory support by the TAH. As a result, investigations continued. Following approval and initial trials of the Jarvik-7 TAH, the Texas Heart Institute used this device as a bridge to transplantation in two patients.

We are currently evaluating the Lapeyre artificial heart in calves and, as a result of these evaluations, believe that this total artificial heart shows great promise for the future. The Lapeyre heart, which incorporates two pumping chambers into one housing, more closely resembles the native heart than previous designs. In this design, the right ventricle partially surrounds the left ventricle (Fig. 9).

Most recently, we have conducted clinical tests of the HeartMate left ventricular assist device (Thermo Cardiosystems, Inc.; Woburn, Massachusetts) in bridge to transplant procedures. Thus far, our results show that we can support patients, even for extended periods of time, until a donor can be located. Furthermore, the HeartMate not only can improve the circulatory status of patients during support, but also can make them more viable transplant candidates.

Designed for intra-abdominal placement, the HeartMate is currently pneumatically powered (Fig. 10). Prior to clinical studies, we conducted 80 bovine experiments, for a cumulative experience of 10 years. Clinical trials began in 1986, at which time we used the device as a

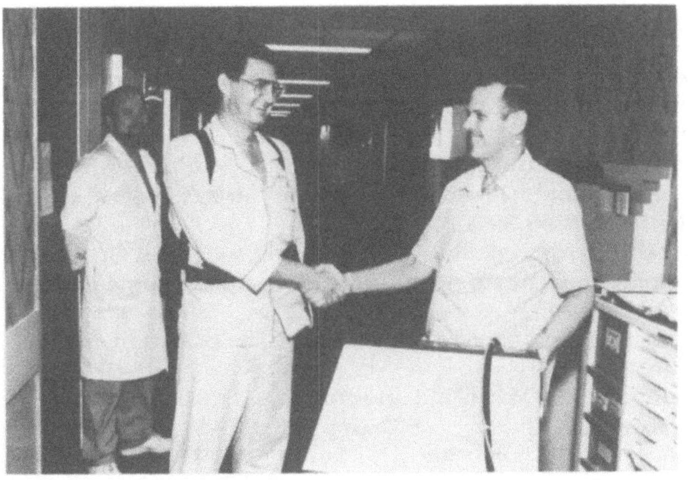

Figure 11. The first patient to undergo successful implantation of the electrical version of the HeartMate (left) shakes the hand of a patient being supported by the pneumatic version of the device.

bridge to transplant in four men. The HeartMate, a pulsatile pump, can provide flows up to 10 L/min. Because of its unique blood-contacting surfaces, anticoagulants such as sodium warfarin and heparin are not required. During the cumulative support time of 90 days in these patients, device performance was excellent, and none of the patients experienced device-related complications. Since then, the pneumatic version of the HeartMate has been used to support an additional 23 patients (November 1991). Recently, we began the first clinical trials of the electrical version of the device. With the electrical device, the patient does not need to be tethered to a large control console, and, thus, is able to move about freely (Fig. 11). Two patients have been supported by the electrical version of the device. No patients have experienced infectious or thromboembolic complications during support. In addition, we have found that pretransplant support with the HeartMate does not necessarily place patients at a higher risk of experiencing postoperative complications, infections, or rejection within the first 6 months after transplant.

The HeartMate offers a good anatomic fit, eliminates the need for anticoagulation, and provides excellent pump performance. Whereas our results have proved the feasibility of providing mechanical circulatory support during prolonged periods in staged cardiac transplantation, they also suggest the feasibility of a permanent, totally implantable cardiac assist device and total artificial heart.

REFERENCES

1. F.M. Sones, E.K. Shirey, W.L. Proudfit, R.N. Westcott: Cine-coronary arteriography. *Circulation* 20:773;1959.

2. J.H. Gibbon: Application of a mechanical heart and lung apparatus to cardiac surgery. *Minn Med* 37:171;1954.
3. D.A. Cooley, A.C. Beall, P. Grondin: Open-heart operations with disposable oxygenators, 5 per cent dextrose prime, and normothermia. *Surgery* 52:713;1962.
4. P. Sergeant, E. Lesaffre, W. Flameng, R. Suy, E. Blackstone: The return of clinically evident ischemia after coronary artery bypass grafting. *Eur J Cardio-thorac Surg* 5:447;1991.
5. D.P. Demikhov: Experimental Transplantation of Vital Organs (authorized translation from the Russian). New York, Consultants Bureau Enterprises, 1962.
6. V.I. Kolesov, L.V. Potashow: Operations on the coronary arteries. *Exp Chir Anaesth* 10:3;1965.
7. A.R. Gruentzig, R.K. Myler, E.S. Hanna, M.I. Turina: Coronary transluminal angioplasty. *Circulation* 55-56(Suppl III):111-84;1977.
8. D.R. Holmes Jr, R.E. Vlietstra, H.C. Smith et al: Restenosis after percutaneous transluminal coronary angioplasty (PTCA): a report from the PTCA Registry of the National Heart, Lung, and Blood Institute. *Am J Cardiol* 53:77C;1984.
9. R.M. Califf, D.F. Fortin, D.J. Frid: Restenosis after coronary angioplasty: an overview. *J Am Coll Cardiol* 17(Suppl B):2B;1991.
10. D.A. Cooley, H.A. Collins, G.C. Morris Jr, D.W. Chapman: Ventricular aneurysm after myocardial infarction: surgical excision with use of temporary cardiopulmonary bypass. *JAMA* 167:557;1958.
11. D.A. Cooley: Ventricular endoaneurysmorrhaphy: results of an improved method of repair. *Texas Heart Institute Journal* 16:72;1989.
12. D.A. Cooley: Repair of the calcified ventricular aneurysm. *Ann Thorac Surg* 49:489;1990.
13. V. Dor, M. Saab, P.Coste et al: Left ventricular aneurysm: a new surgical approach. *Thorac Cardiovasc Surg* 37:11;1989.
14. A.D. Jatene: Left ventricular aneurysmectomy. Resection or reconstruction? *J Thorac Cardiovasc Surg* 50:157;1985.
15. D.A. Cooley, M.T. Ingram: Intravalvular implantation of mitral valve prostheses. *Texas Heart Institute Journal* 14:188;1987.
16. C.W. Lillehei, M.J. Levy, R.C. Bonnabeau: Mitral valve replacement with preservation of papillary muscles and chordae tendineae. *J Thorac Cardiovasc Surg* 47:532;1964.
17. P.A. Spence, C.M. Peniston, T.E. David et al: Toward a better understanding of the etiology of left ventricular dysfunction after mitral valve replacement: An experimental study with possible clinical implications. *Ann Thorac Surg* 41:363;1986.
18. D.E. Hansen, P.D. Cahill, G.C. Derby, D.C. Miller: Relative contributions of the anterior and posterior mitral chordae tendineae to canine global left ventricular systolic function. *J Thorac Cardiovasc Surg* 93:45;1987.
19. D.A. Cooley, J.M. Duncan, D.A. Ott et al: The Texas Heart Institute experience with the St. Jude Medical valve. In D'Alessandro LC, ed. *Heart Surgery*, Rome, Casa Editrice Scientifica Internazionale, 289-296;1987.
20. D.A. Cooley, M.E. DeBakey: Surgical considerations of intrathoracic aneurysms of the aorta and great vessels. *Ann Surg* 135:660;1952.
21. D.A. Cooley, A. Romagnoli, J.D. Milam, M.I. Bossart: A method of preparing woven Dacron grafts to prevent interstitial hemorrhage. Cardiovascular Diseases, Bulletin of the Texas Heart Institute 8:48;1981.
22. S.G. Ablaza, S.C. Ghosh, V.P. Grana: Use of a ringed intraluminal graft in the surgical treatment of dissecting aneurysms of the thoracic aorta. A new technique. *J Thorac Cardiovasc Surg* 76:390;1978.

23. S.L. Lansman, M.A. Ergin, J.D. Galla, M.A. Taylor, R.A. Griepp: Intraluminal graft repair of ascending, arch, descending and thoracoabdominal aortic segments for dissecting and aneurysmal disease: long-term follow-up. Seminars in Thoracic and Cardiovascular Surgery 3:180;1991.
24. D.A. Cooley, D.A. Ott, O.H. Frazier, W.E. Walker: Surgical treatment of aneurysms of the transverse aortic arch: experience with 25 patients using hypothermic techniques. *Ann Thorac Surg* 32:260;1981.
25. J.J. Livesay, D.A. Cooley, J.M. Duncan, D.A. Ott, W.E. Walker, G.J. Reul: Open aortic anastomosis: improved results in the treatment of aneurysms of the aortic arch. *Circulation* 66(suppl I):I-122;1982.
26. R. Elmquist, J. Landegren, S.O. Petterson et al: Artificial pacemaker for treatment of Adams-Stokes syndrome and slow heart rate. *Am Heart J* 65:731;1963.
27. D.A. Ott, A. Garson, D.A. Cooley, D.G. McNamara: Definitive operation for refractory cardiac tachyarrhythmias in children. *J Thorac Cardiovasc Surg* 90:681;1985.
28. P.C. Gillette, A. Garson, J.D. Kugler: Wolff-Parkinson-White syndrome in children: electrophysiologic and pharmacologic characteristics. *Circulation* 60:1487;1979.
29. F. Fontan, E. Baudet: Surgical repair of tricuspid atresia. *Thorax* 26:240;1971.
30. D.B. Doty, J.M. Marvin Jr, R.M. Lauer: Modified Fontan procedure: methods to achieve direct anastomosis of right atrium to pulmonary artery. *J Thorac Cardiovasc Surg* 81:470;1981.
31. G.O. Kreutzer, F.J. Vargas, A.J. Schlichter et al: Atriopulmonary anastomosis. *J Thorac Cardiovasc Surg* 83:427;1982.
32. P. Russo, G.K. Danielson, F.J. Puga et al: Modified Fontan procedure for biventricular hearts with complex forms of double-outlet right ventricle. Circulation 78 (Suppl III);1988.
33. R.A. Jonas, A.R. Castaneda: Modified Fontan procedure: atrial baffle and systemic venous to pulmonary artery anastomotic techniques. *J Cardiac Surg* 3:91;1988.
34. J.E. Mayer Jr, H. Helgason, R.A. Jonas et al: Extending the limits for modified Fontan procedures. *J Thorac Cardiovasc Surg* 92:1021;1986.
35. M.R. de Leval, P. Kilner, M. Gewillig et al: Total cavopulmonary connection: a logical alternative to atriopulmonary connection for complex Fontan operations. *J Thorac Cardiovasc Surg* 96:682;1988.
36. D.A. Cooley, B.K. Sharma, D.E. Lammermeier, G.J. Reul: Modified total cavopulmonary connection: an alternative approach in the presence of left superior vena cava. *Journal of Cardiac Surgery* 5:298;1990.
37. A. Senning: Surgical correction of transposition of the great vessels. *Surgery* 45:966;1959.
38. W.T. Mustard: Successful two-stage correction of transposition of the great vessels. *Surgery* 55:469;1964.
39. W.T. Mustard, H.D. Keith, G.A. Trusler, R. Fowler, L. Kidd: The surgical management of transposition of the great vessels. *J Thorac Cardiovasc Surg* 49:953;1964.
40. M.T. Ingram, L.V. Segesser, D.A. Ott, J.C. Huhta, D.J. Murphy: Senning repair for transposition of the great arteries without patch augmentation of the septum. *J Thorac Cardiovasc Surg* 96:485;1988.
41. A.D. Jatene, V.F. Fontes, P.P. Paulista et al: Anatomical correction of transposition of the great vessels. *J Thorac Cardiovasc Surg* 72:364;1976.
42. Y. Lecompte, L. Zannini, E. Hazan et al: Anatomic correction of transposition of the great arteries: new technique without use of a prosthetic conduit. *J Thorac Cardiovasc Surg* 82:629;1981.

43. G.C. Rastelli, R.B. Wallace, P.A. Ongley: Complete repair of transposition of the great arteries with pulmonary stenosis: a review and report of a case corrected by using a new surgical technique. *Circulation* 39:83;1969.
44. D.A. Cooley, O.H. Frazier, C.T. Van Buren, J.T. Bricker, B. Radovancevic: Cardiac transplantation in an 8-month-old female infant with subendocardial fibroelastosis. *JAMA* 256:1326;1986.
45. C.F. Heck, S.J. Shumway, M.P. Kaye: The Registry of the International Society for Heart Transplantation. *J Heart Transplant* 8:271;1989.
46. D.A. Cooley, D. Liotta, G.L. Hallman et al: Orthotopic cardiac prosthesis for two-staged cardiac replacement. *Am J Cardiol* 24:723;1969.
47. D.A. Cooley, T. Akutsu, J.C. Norman, M.A. Serrato, O.H. Frazier: Total artificial heart in two-staged cardiac transplantation. *Cardiovascular Diseases, Bulletin of the Texas Heart Institute* 8:305;1981.

CARDIAC SURGERY WITHOUT TRANSFUSION: A REAPPRAISAL

Richard K. Spence, M.D.

Department of Surgery
University of Medicine and Dentistry of New Jersey
Robert Wood Johnson School of Medicine
Cooper Hospital/University Medical Center
Camden, New Jersey

INTRODUCTION

In the 1970's, it was not uncommon for patients undergoing open heart surgery to be typed and crossed for 20 or more units of blood. Much of this was used to prime the heart/lung machine; some was transfused directly to the patient. At that time, blood transfusion was regarded as an innocuous procedure with little risk other than an occasional transfusion reaction and the rare case of hepatitis. We have learned much about the dangers of transfusion in cardiac surgery since that time, spurred on by the appearance of AIDS in a number of former patients. The risk of transmitting not only AIDS but also other viruses such as cytomegalovirus and hepatitis has been joined by the potential of immunosuppressing our patients and increasing their susceptibility to infection through transfusion. The need to avoid these complications and to provide a greater margin of safety are compelling reasons to review and revise our transfusion practices. The paragraphs that follow address the progress we have made towards the goal of bloodless cardiac surgery and offer both recommendations for current practice and suggestions for the future.

Is the goal of bloodless cardiac surgery attainable? Clearly, we have made significant progress toward that goal and, in some cases, have reached it. Transfusion requirements in cardiac surgery have declined dramatically over the last decade. Maximum surgical blood ordering schedules based on reviews of large numbers of patients now call for a type and cross of only 3 units of blood for coronary bypass surgery.[1] Accepted indications for transfusion have moved away from reliance on an arbitrarily decided hemoglobin level to consideration of a patient's

Cardiac Surgery: Current Issues, Edited by A.C. Cernaianu
and A.J. DelRossi Plenum Press, New York, 1992

TABLE I. Bloodless cardiac surgery.

Preoperative Measures	
	Check Hgb/Hct early
	Check iron stores
	Check nutritional status
	Limit blood drawing
	Schedule autologous predonation
Intraoperative Measures	
	General principles
	Hemodilution
	Platelet sequestration
	Autotransfusion
	Blood substitutes/alternatives
	Drugs
Postoperative Measures	
	Drugs
	Autotransfusion
	Blood withdrawal
	Nutrition

clinical condition.[2] Transfusions in cardiac surgery are more likely to occur in anemic patients, those over 70 years of age, in emergency cases, and during reoperative surgery.[3] Cooley and colleagues have demonstrated that bloodless cardiac surgery can be performed safely with an acceptable mortality.[4]

The approach to limiting blood transfusion in cardiac surgery can be divided conveniently into preoperative, operative and postoperative activities, with the understanding that there is some overlap in each of these areas. (Table 1) Perhaps the most critical of these is the preoperative period, because failure to act at this time can have a major influence on the amount of homologous blood our patients receive. Specifically, autologous predonation must be considered and arranged early in the preoperative interval.

PREOPERATIVE MEASURES

Autologous predonation has had a significant impact in reducing both the number of patients who receive homologous blood and the number of units transfused. In a study of 271 consecutive patients undergoing elective open heart surgery, Owings and colleagues showed that autologous predonation resulted in homologous transfusion in only 27% of patients.[5] This information is even more compelling given the fact that 82% of the group that did not predonate required homologous transfusion. The amount of homologous blood given to the predonation group was significantly lower, 0.8 ± 1.5 units vs. 3.7 ± 3.6

units. Clearly, autologous predonation can reduce exposure to homologous red cells in the cardiac surgery patient.

Two factors have a significant impact on the success of autologous predonation programs: physician acceptance and sufficient lead time. Unfortunately, many physicians are either unaware of the existence of such programs or are unfamiliar with how to arrange predonation for their patients. A nationwide study of autologous predonation for both cardiac and noncardiac surgery estimated that only 10% of eligible patients actually gave blood before surgery.[6] Toy and associates suggested that this may be due in part to physicians resistance because of perceived inconvenience for both themselves and their patients. Goodnough found that predonation was not offered to nay open-heart patients in one of two hospitals he studied in spite of the fact that the institution had active autologous program.[7]

In addition to physician cooperation, successful predonation requires a lead time of one month if patients are to donate adequate amounts of blood before admission and still have an acceptable hematocrit. From one to six units, or an average of 3 units of red cells can be donated in this amount of time.[5] The administration of erythropoietin can increase this average by stimulating red cell mass recovery. Goodnough's study of the effect of erythropoietin on predonation in elective orthopedic surgical patients demonstrated a 41% red cell volume per patient increased in treated patients.[8] This group donated an average of 5.4 units of blood as compared to 4.1 units for the control group while maintaining comparable hematocrits.

What are the limitations for autologous predonation of blood aside from the lead time required? Patients must have an hematocrit of 34% or higher. Using this limitation, 15 to 20% of patients will be unable to donate.[5] The ability to donate may be limited by disease or medications, especially iron-deficiency anemia. This diagnosis can be made easily by checking red cell indices along with the hematocrit to look for the characteristic hypochromic, microcytic anemia. Treatment with oral iron therapy, 325 mg of ferrous sulfate or gluconate by mouth, three times a day, should be started early and continued through the perioperative period. Even the patient without iron-deficiency anemia will benefit from oral iron replacement to permit rapid recovery of the red cell mass after phlebotomy. This is especially true in the patient on erythropoietin, who will *become* iron deficient rapidly if iron utilized is not replaced. Women tend to be more iron-deficient than men and donate on average on unit less.[5]

Since the hematocrit usually recovers in less than one week after phlebotomy, patients can donate safely up to 72 hours before admission. The usual amount of blood drawn at one time is 500 ml. In the cardiac patient, a margin of safety is added by slowly infusing equal volumes of saline during phlebotomy to prevent sudden drops in blood pressure. Studies of standard blood donors over the age of 65 years have shown that the process is both safe and feasible.[9] The mean age of autologous donors in Owings group was 63.3 years.[5] Therefore, age alone is not a contraindication to autologous donation. Severity of disease, specifically critical aortic stenosis and unstable angina requiring hospitalization, may prevent patients from giving blood before surgery.

We must make a major change in our thinking during preoperative evaluations if we are to be successful in reducing homologous blood transfusion in cardiac surgery. Our focus must be broadened to include not only the patient's cardiac disease and catheterization studies, but also his/her hematologic status and accompanying diseases. Unfortunately, many cardiac surgeons see patients late in the preoperative period and have little time to initiate successful predonation. In this case, discussions with referring cardiologists are essential to assure that patients begin donating blood early enough to make the precess worthwhile.

INTRAOPERATIVE MEASURES

Principles of avoiding and controlling blood loss during surgery are applicable to all types of procedures, not just cardiac operations. We have found that scoring the skin with the scalpel, then continuing the incision with electrocautery has helped minimize troublesome subcutaneous bleeding. Although blood loss at this point is usually minimal, hypertensive patients can bleed heavily from subcutaneous vessels. Who among us has not found wound drapes or towels saturated from a slow skin ooze at the end of a case? Early attention to skin vessels can prevent unsuspected blood loss. In our hands, the use of electrocautery has not lead to increased infections and has not interfered with wound healing.

Cautery can be used successfully when making a median sternotomy and in dissecting out internal mammary arteries. Careful dissection along bloodless planes helps prevent unexpected blood loss. Where this is not possible or when bleeding is encountered, it should be stopped immediately. We have been particularly careful about observing this rule in our Jehovah's Witness patients in whom any blood lost is blood that cannot be replaced. The most frequent sites of slow bleeding in open heart surgery are the superior mediastinum and the internal mammary artery bed. Bleeding from these sites usually can be controlled by cautery or suture ligation.

The days of priming the heart/lung machine with whole blood are gone. Most cardiac surgeons and perfusionists use a crystalloid prime, both to eliminate blood product exposure and to provide for hemodilution. As the patient goes on bypass, the hematocrit gradually is reduced to 20-25% to attain isovolemic hemodilution. Isovolemic hemodilution offers the advantage of improved microcirculatory flow secondary to decreased blood viscosity. In addition, blood is diluted so fewer red cells are lost. Most patients tolerate hemodilution without difficulties and recover well postoperatively if ventricular function is normal.[10]

Decreases in colloid osmotic pressure may present a problem postoperatively in the form of edema for some patients if a crystalloid prime is used. This may be overcome in part by using artificial colloids such as dextran or hydroxyethyl starch. Oxygen carrying blood substitutes have not yet become useful in this setting. Hemodilution frequently is accompanied by hypothermia to decrease oxygen utilization.

Cardiopulmonary bypass requires systemic anticoagulation using heparin. Activated clotting times should be prolonged from a normal range of 80 to 130 seconds to 400 seconds to prevent coagulation in the heart/lung machine. Frequent monitoring and reversal of the heparin effect with protamine at the conclusion of the procedure can prevent most problems from heparin-induced bleeding. Although both hemodilution and hypothermia may interfere with clotting mechanisms, the effect is minimal.

A more serious problem and cause of undesirable postoperative bleeding is platelet dysfunction, Platelets are rapidly consumed during the first few minutes on bypass and surface glycoproteins are activated. Contact with the foreign surface of the pump appears to affect the GpIIb/IIIa adhesive protein system, leading to a qualitative, as well as a quantitative defect. The amount of time on bypass correlates directly with postoperative bleeding. Patients on bypass for more than two hours (120 minutes) have higher transfusion requirements than those with shorter exposures.[3]

Several investigators have developed an approach to this problem using intraoperative autotransfusion techniques combined with hemodilution.[11] Five hundred milliliters of blood are removed via a central venous catheter while crystalloid is infused simultaneously, resulting in initial hemodilution. The blood is separated into a red cell pack and platelet-rich plasma using a standard, centrifuge driven autotransfusion device. The red cells can be given as needed at any time in the case. The platelet-rich plasma is returned following cessation of bypass and heparin reversal. With this approach, a portion of the patient's clotting factors and platelets can avoid exposure to both heparin and the artificial surface of the heart/lung machine. Both blood loss and transfusion need have been decreased with this technique, the former by 10-35% and the latter by 60-65%. Autologous, predonated blood can be treated in a similar way although differing shelf lives and storage requirements for blood components limit its usefulness.

Autotransfusion using the systems that collect, wash and transfuse shed blood during surgery are familiar to most cardiac surgeons. Any blood lost during the operation should be collected using one of these systems. Similarly, any blood remaining in the pump after bypass should be processed and reinfused. Washing destroys some red cells but it also eliminates unwanted debris and coagulation products that may have been generated during blood contact with the heart-lung machine surfaces. Filtering can reduce even further the number of potentially harmful white cell complexes and coagulation byproducts that the patient receives.

Pharmacologic manipulation of blood loss holds promise for the future of cardiac surgery. Initial experience has been gained with two drugs, desmopressin and aprotinin. Desmopressin, frequently abbreviated as DDAVP, is 1-deamino-8-D-arginine vasopressin. Unlike vasopressin, it has little pressor effect, but it does not act as an antidiuretic. Its main role in minimizing bleeding during cardiac surgery derives from its ability to elevate both Factor VIII and Factor VIII:vonWillebrand's Factor two to three fold over normal levels. DDAVP can add a significant advantage in selected patients, e.g., hemophiliacs, who have low factor VIII levels. However, its role in cardiac surgical patients is controversial. Some investigators believe that DDAVP is contraindicated in patients with a history of myocardial infarction or angina.[12]

The optimal dose of DDAVP in platelet dysfunction in noncardiac surgery is 0.3 micrograms per kilogram. Efficacy trials have produced mixed results. Both Czer and Salzman described decreases in blood loss and transfusion need following open heart surgery when DDAVP was administered.[12,13] However, in similar studies, Rocha and Hackmann showed no change in either of these parameters.[14,15] At the present time, we do not recommend routine use of DDAVP in cardiac surgical patients. Further studies are needed to clarify its effect in this setting.

Aprotinin, or Trasylol, is a serine proteinase inhibitor that has been used most often in the past to treat pancreatitis. The mechanism by which it reduces bleeding is uncertain, but it is thought to be mediated through either its inhibition of kallikrein and/or plasmin or its preservation of platelet adhesion membrane receptors during cardiopulmonary bypass. Trials in over 200 open-heart patients have shown that Aprotinin reduces both blood loss and transfusion need, the former by 45-80% and the latter by up to 75% when compared to control groups.[16-18] In addition, vanOeveren and colleagues have shown that platelet adhesiveness is maintained when Aprotinin is given to patients treated with aspirin before coronary bypass surgery.[19] In their randomized study of 60 patients, bleeding time was 30% lower and blood loss was reduced significantly.

Unfortunately, Aprotinin is not without side effects and potential risk. The drug must be given intravenously in large amounts and frequently causes hypotension, which can vary in severity. The drug is eliminated via the kidney and has a tendency to accumulate in the proximal tubule where it may produce acute tubular necrosis. Although Aprotinin appears to offer significant advantages to the cardiac surgeon, its toxicity and potential for harm must be considered seriously before it is used routinely.

We have included fibrin glue in this discussion of drug therapy in cardiac surgery although it is not a pharmacologic agent per se. Fibrin glue is made by reacting a source of fibrinogen, either fresh frozen plasma or cryoprecipitate, with thrombin to produce fibrin. The material adheres well to biological surfaces and has been shown to be effective in controlling bleeding from solid organs such as the liver and spleen.[20] It could be of help in preventing difficult bleeding from the sternum or in reoperative cardiac cases. Fibrin glue "sets up" quickly and adheres firmly, so mixing must be done at the site of application. Autologous plasma should be used rather than homologous, as has been done in most reported cases, if blood product exposure is to be avoided.

Blood substitutes have yet to play a major role in cardiac surgery, in spite of their potential. Perfluorocarbon emulsions, such as Fluosol, have demonstrated their ability to dissolve oxygen and directly increase oxygen delivery in both animal studies and human trials.[21] Fluosol is currently available on the market for use in conjunction with coronary angioplasty because it protects myocardium distal to the inflated balloon. Fluosol also appears to be effective in limiting myocardial reperfusion injury in models where infusions were given either before or after acute coronary artery occlusion.[22] Buckberg and his group have evaluated Fluosol as a cardioplegic agent in a dog model.[23] He found that Fluosol cardioplegia was superior to both normal blood reperfusion and to initial cardioplegia using either colloid or crystalloid. However, its ability to limit damage from reperfusion, although considerable, was inferior to blood cardioplegia. Buckberg suggests that changes in perfluorocarbon formulations such as the addition of oxygen free radical scavengers may improve their cardioplegic capabilities. Second generation perfluorocarbons with higher weight per unit volume concentrations and, therefore, more oxygen carrying capacity, should be evaluated for use not only as cardioplegic agents but as pump primes.

Stroma-free hemoglobin (SFH) solutions with hemoglobin concentrations of 14 gm/dl have been shown to be capable of sustaining life in essentially asanguinous animals. However, initial clinical trials were halted after reactions occurred in two patients. The reasons for the reactions are unknown and require further investigation. SFH has been used successfully as a cardioplegic agent in the laboratory and holds promise for the future, once problems with toxicity and reactions have been solved.[24]

Whereas most cardiac surgeons have begun to limit their use of red blood cell transfusion to prevent disease transmission, it would appear that many have failed to realize that fresh frozen plasma (FFP) is as potentially dangerous as blood. Fresh frozen plasma should not be infused to increase volume or to replace presumably absent clotting factors. The surgeon is obliged to demonstrate by direct measurement that clotting factors are abnormally low before infusing FFP and thereby exposing his patient to risk. Martinowitz and colleagues recently demonstrated that infusion of FFP in open heart patients did not decrease bleeding time or improve platelet function when compared to fresh, whole blood.[25] We believe that FFP infusions should be abandoned in most patients and replaced by infusions of autologous platelet-rich plasma. Although heat-treated albumin carries little known risk of disease transmission, the surgeon who wishes to remain completely blood-free, e.g., in a Jehovah's Witness, can substitute pentastarch for albumin without fear of clotting abnormalities or disturbances in cardiopulmonary hemodynamics.[26]

POSTOPERATIVE MEASURES

Postoperative measures are, by and large, continuations of those steps that have been taken both pre- and intraoperatively to limit the need for homologous transfusion. These may include continuation of nutritional support, iron therapy and erythropoietin to stimulate red cell production. DDAVP and Aprotinin can be used in the postoperative setting to control blood loss, but they should not be substitutes for early re-exploration in the actively bleeding patient.

Postoperative autotransfusion of shed mediastinal blood has been shown to be of significant benefit in reducing the need for homologous transfusion by as much as 50%.[27] Disposable, sterile systems that collect blood for reinfusion are readily available in most ICUs. They are limited by the fact that considerable amounts of debris, clotted blood, and free hemoglobin accumulate in a short period of time. Either washing or filtering can deliver a purer product and eliminate some of the concerns over infusion potentially harmful substances. Once again, reliance on the ability to reinfuse shed mediastinal blood should not prevent the surgeon from returning a patient to the operating room if re-exploration is indicated.

Perhaps the biggest transfusion-related problem the cardiac surgeon faces in the postoperative period is the tendency in the ICU, however well-meaning, to bleed his patient for laboratory studies. Now that postoperative hemoglobin levels of 7, 8 or 9 gm/dl are routinely accepted, few patients can tolerate repeated blood sampling. The amount of blood that can be withdrawn should not be underestimated. Smoller and Kruskall measured daily blood losses from phlebotomy of 41.5 ml in ICU patients.[28] This amounts to approximately a one unit blood loss per week.

Blood sampling in the ICU should be limited to only essential studies. We use pediatric collection tubes routinely in our Jehovah's Witness patients and return blood from arterial and central flushes. The adoption of similar practices can prevent significant iatrogenic blood loss, especially in complicated patients who spend more than one or two days in the ICU.

In this brief overview, we have addressed preoperative, operative and postoperative measures than can be employed to reduce the need for homologous blood transfusion in open heart patients. These range from currently used techniques of autotransfusion and hemodilution to promising new pharmacologic therapies designed to prevent bleeding, restore the red cell mass, or replace blood entirely. Although it is highly improbable that homologous blood transfusion will be eliminated completely from cardiac surgery, by using these approaches and therapies, bloodless cardiac surgery should be possible in the majority of patients.

REFERENCES

1. T.A. Lowery, J.A. Clark: Successful implementation of a maximum surgical blood ordering schedule. *J Med Assos GA* 78-3:155-8;1989.
2. R.K. Spence: The status of bloodless surgery. *Transf Med Rev* Vol 4:274-86;1991.
3. D.M. Cosgrove, F.D. Loop, B.N. Lytle, et al: Determinants of blood utilization during myocardial revascularization. *Ann Thorac Surg* 40:380-84;1985.
4. D.A. Ott, D.A. Cooley: Cardiovascular surgery in Jehovah's Witnesses. *JAMA* 238(12):1256-8;1977.
5. D.V. Owings, M.S. Kruskall, R.L. Thurer, et al: Autologous blood donations prior to elective cardiac surgery. *JAMA* 262:1963;1968.
6. PTCY Toy, R.G. Strauss, L.G. Stehling, et al: Predeposited autologous blood for elective surgery: A national multicenter study. *N Engl J Med* 316(9):517-520;1987.
7. L.T. Goodnough, M.F.M. Johnston, PTCY Toy, et al: The variability of transfusion practice in coronary artery bypass surgery. *JAMA* 265(1):86-90;1991.
8. L.T. Goodnough: Erythropoietin as a pharmacologic alternative to blood transfusion in the surgical patient. *Transf Med Rev* 4:288-296;1990.
9. J. Pindyck, J. Avorn, M. Kuriyan, et al: Blood donation by the elderly: Clinical and policy decisions. *JAMA* 257:1186-1188;1987.
10. P.G. Robertie, G.P. Grvalee: Safe limits of isovolemic hemodilution and recommendations for erythrocyte transfusion. *Int Anesthesiol Clin* 28:197-204;1990.
11. A.J. DelRossi, A.C. Cernaianu, R.A. Vertrees, et al: Platelet-rich plasma reduces postoperative blood loss after cardiopulmonary bypass. *J Thorac Cardiovasc Surg* 100:281-286;1990.
12. E.W. Salzman, M.J. Weinstein, R.M. Weintraub, et al: Treatment with desmopressin acetate to reduce blood loss after cardiac surgery: A double blind randomized trial. *N Engl J Med* 314:1402-1406;1986.
13. L.S.C. Czer, T.M. Bateman, R.J. Gray, et al: Treatment of severe platelet dysfunction and hemorrhage after cardiopulmonary bypass: Reduction in blood product usage with desmopressin. *J Am Coll Cardiol* 9:1139-1147;1987.
14. E. Rocha, R. Llorens, J.A. Paramo, et al: Does desmopressin acetate reduce blood loss after surgery in patients on cardiopulmonary bypass? *Circulation* 77:1319-1323;1988.
15. T. Hackman, R.D. Gascoyne, S.C. Naiman, et al: A trial of desmopressin (1-desamino-8-D-arginine-vasopressin) to reduce blood loss in uncomplicated cardiac surgery. *N Engl J Med* 321:1437-1443;1989.
16. D. Royston, B.P. Bidstrup, K.M. Taylor, et al: Effect of aprotinin on need for transfusion after repeat open heart surgery. *Lancet* 2:1289-1291;1987.
17. B.P. Bidstrup, D. Royston, R.N. Sapsford, et al: Reduction in blood loss after cardiopulmonary bypass using high dose aprotinin (Trasylol): Studies in patients undergoing aortocoronary bypass surgery, reoperations and valve replacement for endocarditis. *J Thorac Cardiovasc Surg* 97:364-372;1989.
18. G. Fraedrich G, C. Weber, H. Engler, et al: Benefits and risks of aprotinin in open heart surgery. *J Cardiovasc Surg* 31:44;1990.

19. W. Van Oeveren, N.J. Jansen, B.P. Bidstrup, et al: Effects of aprotinin on hemostatic mechanism during cardiopulmonary bypass. *Ann Thorac Surg* 44:640-645;1987.
20. H.B. Kram, R.C. Nathan, F.J. Stafford, et al: Fibrin glue achieves hemostasis in patients with coagulation disorders. *Arch Surg* 124:385-387;1989.
21. R.K. Spence, S. McCoy, J. Costabile, et al: Fluosol DA-20% in the treatment of severe anemia: Randomized, controlled study of 46 patients. *Crit Care Med* 18:1227-1230;1990.
22. R.K. Spence: Fluosol and the heart. *Cardiac Chron* 5(1):1-6; 1991.
23. C. Acar, M.T. Partington, G.D. Buckberg: Studies of controlled reperfusion after ischemia. *J Thorac Cardiovasc Surg* 101:284-293;1991.
24. T.I. Pristoupil, M. Vrana, J. Havlickova, et al: Hemoglobin solutions in experimental cardioplegia. *Int J Artif Organs* 12(10):668-672;1989.
25. U. Martiniwitz, D.A. Goor, B. Ramot, et al: Is transfusion of fresh plasma after cardiac operations indicate? *J Thorac Cardiovasc Surg* 100:92-98;1990.
26. M.J. London, J.S. Ho, J.K. Treidman, et al: A randomized clinical trial of 10% pentastarch (low molecular weight hydroxyethyl starch) versus 5% albumin for plasma volume expansion after cardiac operations. *J Thorac Cardiovasc Surg* 97:785-797;1989.
27. A. Adan, A. Brutel de le Riviere, F. Haas, et al: Autotransfusion of drained mediastinal blood after cardiac surgery: A reappraisal. *Thorac Cardiovasc Surgeon* 36:10-14;1988.
28. B.R. Smoller, M.S. Kruskall: Phlebotomy for diagnostic laboratory tests in adults: Pattern of use and effect on transfusion requirements. *N Engl J Med* 314:1233-1235;1986.

PHYSIOLOGY OF BLOOD FLOW DURING CARDIOPULMONARY PERFUSION

Roger A. Vertrees, B.A., C.C.P. and
Louis Brownstein, B.A., C.C.P.

Department of Surgery, Division of Cardiothoracic Surgery
School of Cardiovascular Perfusion
University of Medicine and Dentistry of New Jersey
Robert Wood Johnson Medical School at Camden
Cooper Hospital/University Medical Center
Camden, New Jersey

The purpose of this chapter is to identify the factors that play determinant roles in affecting the blood flow during cardiopulmonary bypass (CPB). Under normal physiological conditions, blood is contained within the circulatory system which is a closed circuit. The system is influenced by many factors which contribute to the normal blood rheology. These factors will be presented as the initial step of this discussion.

During cardiovascular perfusion there are many factors influencing the circulatory system. CPB creates an open and increased circulatory space where "non-physiological events" are taking place. These alterations of homeostasis induced by CPB will be discussed later in this chapter.

FACTORS AFFECTING BLOOD FLOW

Diffusion is the fundamental transport mechanism in living organisms and occurs because all molecules are in continuous, random, thermal motion. Molecules collide and bounce off each other as they come into contact. Consequently, the more densely packed, the more the number of collisions. The result of each collision is a change in direction of the colliding molecules. When the molecules' concentration is reduced, the number of collisions decreases with resultant less

Cardiac Surgery: Current Issues, Edited by A.C. Cernaianu
and A.J. DelRossi Plenum Press, New York, 1992

change of direction. This allows the molecules to spread out into the environment, this continues until the molecules achieve the same concentration anywhere in the solution. The overall result of this continued process allows for a spread from a region with higher concentration to a region with low concentration and continues until the system reaches a state of equilibrium; The advantage of diffusion is that it requires no energy in the presence of a permeable membrane. However, the disadvantage of diffusion is, that it's effectiveness is inversely proportional to the distance of transportation, ceasing to become an effective transport mechanism at transfer distances greater than 1 mm. Since most biological substrates should be transported at a greater distance than 1 mm, a network of vessels has evolved.

In order for the body to use the diffusion mechanism, the internal environment must be brought into close proximity with millions of cells. This is accomplished by a network of vessels that constantly maintain a concentration gradient within the vessels for electrolytes and metabolic substances. Should the maintenance of the gradient disappear, the diffusion cannot take place. The exchange transport system, via the vessels, continually provides a supply of nutrients and chemicals thereby maintaining the required concentration gradient necessary for metabolism.[1]

Blood, which is a viscous fluid, is composed of a cellular compartment, and plasma. Blood is characterized by *viscosity*, which depends on the percentage of the volume occupied by the blood cells. Viscosity may influence the fluid motion by ameliorating the sudden changes in velocity due to acceleration. Approximately 99% of the cellular compartment is composed of red cells, The white blood cells contribute very little to the physical properties of the blood. The hematocrit (Hct), which represents the red cell concentration is approximately 42% for the normal male and about 38% for the normal female.

Viscosity is directly proportional to hematocrit and other blood components.[2,3] Blood has a viscosity of three times that of water which means that it would require much more pressure to move it through a tube than it would water. The viscosity is directly influenced by the number and types of molecules present in the fluid. However, this is not a linear relationship. i.e., when the hematocrit is 60-70%, the viscosity may be 10 fold that of water.

Blood behaves as a pure liquid in vessels whose radius is greater than 1 mm. The Fahraeus-Lindqvist factor defines this arrangement as an organized alignment of red cells moving through vessels with diameters less than 1.5 mm, one cell at a time, resulting in a reduction of it's viscous resistance. This effect reduces the viscous resistance that would result from contact with the vessel wall and from the random arrangement of cells within the vessel. The elasticity of the red cell membrane allows for a change in shape that facilitates passage through these small vessels.[4] Plasma, an acellular environment containing 7% protein, consists of albumin, globulins and fibrinogen and exerts an insignificant effect on the blood's overall viscosity[5]. Plasma acts as a lubricant between the cells and the vessel walls, thus reducing the viscosity to approximately half. There are two counter-forces occurring that will probably cancel out the above effects. Initially, as the velocity of flow decreases because of the small vessel size, red cell aggregation, and a red cell-vessel wall adherence can effectively increase the viscosity by as much as ten times. In small vessels, cell nuclei may protrude into the vessel lumen with the result that blood flow resulting in stagnation or blockage of the blood flow for a short period of time. Occasionally, at this level blood flow may become affected by the presence of the large amorphous white blood cells.

CHARACTERISTICS OF BLOOD FLOW

The movement of blood involves the *potential energy* (blood pressure), and the *kinetic energy* (flow). Both forms of energy are readily converted from one to the other. Blood flow is determined by the pressure difference between both ends of the vessel segment, and the resistance to flow. According to Ohm's Law:

$$Q = dP/R$$

where Q = blood flow, dP = pressure differential, and R = resistance.

The preceding formula defines that blood flow is proportional to the pressure difference and inversely proportional to resistance. This relationship shows that blood flow will decrease as the resistance increases if the pressure remains constant, or as the pressure decreases, either the resistance increases or the flow increases, or possibly, both parameters may increase.[6]

TYPES OF FLOW

An understanding of the term *velocity* is essential to the concept of blood flow during CPB . Output, whether as cardiac output, or pump output is the volume of blood pumped in one minute. Pump output (amount blood displaced) is different from blood flow velocity (rate of blood flow) because the velocity profile within the tube (vessel) is not flat. If this profile was flat, this would imply a constant velocity across the lumen of the vessel. Then pump output would be exactly equal to the velocity (V_{AVE}) multiplied by the cross sectional area (A) of the tube (vessel).[6]

$$Q = A \cdot V_{AVE}$$

Cardiac output, perfusion pump output and blood flow velocity are not equal because the velocity profile across the vessel lumen is not flat, but parabolic. The parabolic interface implies that a variable velocity exists within the vessel. The velocity profile is defined as the interface that exists as blood is propelled through a tube and results from the friction between the fluid and vessel wall. When the heart beats, the roller compresses the tubing, or tangential outflow from a centrifugal pump occurs, the blood flow is directly affected.

When blood flow is steady through a long, smooth vessel, it flows in streamlines.[7] Each layer of blood remains at the same distance from the wall and travels at approximately the same rate with the particles farthest away from the wall traveling the fastest. The overall effect is a laminar or streamline blood flow. Because of friction, causing adherence to the vessel wall, these molecules which contact the vessel wall will have a velocity of zero. The next layer of molecules then slips over this previous layer, which serves as ball bearings, allowing each successive layer to travel under conditions of less friction and greater velocity. Since vessels are cylindrical, the point furthest from the wall is also the point that is located in the center of the vessel, i.e., the point of greatest blood flow velocity.

The second characteristic of blood flow is *turbulence* and occurs as the rate of blood flow becomes too great for the vessel. According to Nelkin[8], ..."when a fluid flows rapidly, it's flow pattern typically exhibits a subtle mixture of order and chaos, and it is this structured chaotic fluid motion that we refer to as turbulence". Turbulence is characterized by random movement of blood throughout the vessel, continually developing secondary flow elements, eddy currents and whorls. As discrimination of flow ceases because of the presence of these secondary flow elements, the velocity profile flattens out. The flatter the profile, the greater becomes the effects of viscous friction which increases the overall resistance to blood flow. It is much more difficult for blood to travel the vessel if turbulence is present as opposed to laminar flow conditions. Turbulence results in an increase in the resistance due to contact of the blood to the vessel wall (friction), and an increase in the resistance due to an "increase" in viscosity. Prediction of turbulence is calculated by the following equation:[9]

$$R_e = V \cdot d \cdot p/\eta$$

[V = velocity, d = diameter of vessel, p = the density, η = viscosity].

Osborne Reynolds discovered about 100 years ago that higher viscosity in a fluid opposes turbulence, whereas higher density makes turbulence more likely[10]. At a high Reynolds number (2000 units), turbulence occurs even in the straight portions of vessels whereas at a far lesser number (200-400 units) it may occur only at some branch points. As the Reynold's number approaches 1,000, turbulence will generally occur in the branch points of most vessels. This number is surpassed in most larger arteries, therefore there is always some turbulent flow in the branches of these vessels.[11] During periods of rapid ventricular ejection, the Reynold's number can rise to several thousand which will cause considerable turbulence in the proximal aorta and pulmonary artery. There is evidence that the Reynold's concept may be inaccurate when applied to pulsatile flow.

As the flow rate increases, the laminar flow velocity profile becomes unstable and secondary flow patterns develop which result in turbulent flow. Once this occurs, the flow rate must be reduced in order to resume laminar flow (hysteresis effect). If an obstruction occurs in an artery, the volume flow will be constant. As the cross-sectional area decreases, an increase in velocity results that may precipitate turbulence and additional workload is needed in order to effectively perfuse the areas distal to the obstruction. This results in a reduction in the volume of blood moved past the point of obstruction.

BLOOD PRESSURE

Another important component of blood flow is *pressure* which is defined by Guyton[12] as "...the force exerted by the blood against any unit area of the vessel wall,..." and results from the movement of blood. The heart is a pulsatile pump which produces in a normal, healthy adult a systolic pressure of 120 mmHg, a diastolic pressure of 80 mmHg, and a pressure difference or pulse pressure of 40 mmHg.

The tracing of the normal pressure wave displays some points of interest. The upstroke of the pressure wave is commonly referred to as dp/dt representing the period of rapid ventricular ejection of blood from the ventricle. It represents the point in time when blood is being accelerated. Peak systole (systolic blood pressure) occurs at the summit of the curve, lasting for 0.2 to 0.3 seconds. The dicrotic notch indicating the aortic valve closure follows and indicates a momentary reversal of blood flow before the steady decline of pressure back to the diastolic level which completes the cycle.

Since the vessel walls are elastic, the area of the vessel lumen increases when the heart ejects blood into the aorta, and decreases during diastole, therefore the aorta becomes a "reservoir" for this ejected blood. This reservoir effect has in essence "smoothed" the heart's acceleration of blood. The majority of peripheral perfusion as well as coronary perfusion takes place during diastole. The pulse pressure becomes dampened as it progresses through the vascular system becoming almost absent in the capillaries as a result of the inertial forces of the moving blood and the compliance of the vessel. As flow progresses through the aorta, it goes from an area of great compliance - *distensibility*, and slow transmission - *large volume*, to vessels of less compliance and quickened transmission (arteries) and from here through the arterioles to the capillaries. In normal conditions it takes about 100 milliseconds for the pulse wave to travel from the ascending aorta to the femoral artery and it depends on the aortic compliance. As flow progresses down the aorta, the diastolic flow increases, causing a delay in the propagation of the pressure and flow pulses. In the peripheral arteries, when they are distended, the pulse pressure encounters a rapidly decreasing compliance, which makes it difficult for the pressure pulse to travel any further. And in the small narrow arteries the pulse wave is reflected back, which further impedes forward progress causing still more dampening of the pulse pressure wave's contours. By the time they reach the capillaries, the pulse pressures often average 1 mmHg.

According to Guyton[13], "...the velocity of transmission of the pulse pressure is much greater than the actual velocity of the blood flow itself." The energy present in the pulse wave is dissipated into the peripheral circulation helping to maintain capillary performance and diffusion gradients. Shepard and Riedel[14] reports that pulsatile flow contains 2.3 times as much energy as does non-pulsatile flow under the same conditions. It is considered that the dispersed energy resulting from pulsatile flow is responsible for maintaining the arteriolar vasomotor tone and total vascular resistance. The transfer of kinetic energy rather than the mean arterial pressure is of greater importance in keeping capillary beds open, lymph flowing, and preventing edema formation.

RESISTANCE

Resistance is defined as the impediment to blood flow in the vessel. In order to understand the concept of resistance, it's relationship to blood flow needs to be examined.

Conductance is a measure of the blood flow through a vessel for a given pressure difference. Conductance which is directly proportional to the diameter of the vessel can cause tremendous changes in the ability of the vessel to transport blood. In laminar flow vessels, the farthest molecule from the walls travel the fastest, consequently, the shorter the transit time becomes. Thus, the result is an increased amount of blood volume to pass a fixed point in the larger vessel. Conductance is inversely proportional to resistance, therefore a vessel which holds more blood offers increasingly less resistance because the molecules become more distantly removed from the vessel walls. According to Poiseuille's Law, blood flow is determined by:

$$Q = \pi \,.\, dP \,.\, r^4/8\eta l$$

where dP = change in pressure, r = radius, η = viscosity and l = length of segment.

It should be noted that resistance is directly proportional to the fourth power of the radius.[15]

The total resistance (R_T) of the vessels in the tissue bed can be calculated as follows:

$$R_T = \frac{1}{1/R_1 + 1/R_2 + 1/R_3 \ldots /R_X}$$

One can imply that the total resistance offered by a tissue bed is less than the resistance of each one of the vessels. Since all the blood did not go through one vessel as it went through the organ, the resistance of each individual vessel would be greater than the resistance of the organ as a whole.

The resistance of vessels in series can be calculated by the following equation:

$$R_T = R_1 + R_2 + \ldots..R_x$$

where R_T is equal to the sum of individual resistances. This system has limited application in the body but significant implications for the perfusionist.

An increase in arterial pressure causes a proportional increase in blood flow through various tissues of the body. An increase in the arterial pressure not only increases the force that pushes blood throughout the vessel, but it also distends the vessel, decreasing it's resistance. Blood flow ceases completely even in situations when a small amount of pressure still remains resulting in a fall in arterial pressure and a decrease in the degree of vessel walls distension. At the point where the pressure inside the vessel can no longer surpass the vessel wall muscle tone, the vessel closes. This point is called the critical closing pressure and is defined by the Law of Laplace which states that the circumferential force tending to stretch the muscle fibers in the vessel wall is proportional to the diameter of the vessel times the pressure inside of the vessel:

$$F = DxP$$

Therefore, as the pressure in the vessel falls there is double reason for the diameter to decrease. First, the decrease in pressure causes a collapse of the vessel, and second, the decreased diameter reduces the force of stretch causing even further decrease in the diameter of the vessel. Another reason for the cessation of blood flow at low arterial pressure is a tendency for the blood cells to adhere to the arterioles and capillaries wall.

ARCHITECTURE OF THE VASCULAR SYSTEM

The metabolism occurs in the intracellular environment. Nutrients are transported to the cell from the vascular system by diffusion. The designs of the vascular system play an integral role in determining the physical distribution of blood. The system has evolved as a transport mechanism for metabolic nutrients and removal of waste.

In order to reach the individual cells from the large vessels, extremely narrow vessels have developed. When blood travels these narrow vessels, a high energy cost is imposed on the system. As mentioned previously, viscosity is a function of the magnitude of the axial velocity and the radius of the vessel, and determines the amount of sheer stress on the vessel wall.

In referring back to the parabolic interface that is produced by blood flow, it is noted that as blood flows through a vessel the layer of molecules contacting the vessel wall exerts a force on the vessel wall. This force is equal and opposite in direction to viscous friction and is called *sheer stress.* A force tending to pull the vessel wall in the downstream direction is created. The shear stress is resistant to the deformation of the fluid by out side factors. In this situation, the product of friction is efficiency loss. The frictional forces cause an efficiency loss which is manifested as heat. Therefore, energy release (heat) is the price paid whenever a fluid moves through a vessel and is one of the major contributors to the maintenance of the body's thermal status.

In a recent article by LaBarbera[16] four principles of vascular architecture are discussed. The author noted, that it takes a great deal more energy to move a fluid through a narrow vessel (peripheral tissue) than through a wide one (core). This can be redefined as *Principle 1.* "...when a biologically relevant physical transfer process is limited to small spacial scales and local depletion of a necessary resource is threatened, bulk flow and other fluids will be utilized for long distance transport of that resource." (Poiseuille's Law has already identified the fact that more energy will be needed to flow fluid through a narrow pipe than through a wide one).

Principle 2 states that "....energy considerations dictate that fluid transport systems utilize both large and small vessels." Small vessels exist at exchange sites and are permeable, whereas all long distance transport occurs in large compliant vessels. The most energy efficient way to build a fluid transport system is to combine both narrow and wide vessels. A narrow vessel can reach the individual cell, with nutrient rich blood traveling very slow, generating heat as it perfuses the transfer sites. The wide vessels can deliver fluids to the narrow vessels over long distances, retaining much in the way of potential energy and nutrient concentration. In the human circulatory system, the aorta is approximately 60 cm long with a radius of 1.25 cm. The vessel delivers blood to the capillaries which serve as the transfer sites and are only about one millimeter long and 4 micrometers in radius. Principle 2 establishes another set of concepts related to the vascular system. As a certain volume of blood enters one end of a vessel segment it must exit the other, i.e., the distal opening should be smaller than the proximal one, therefore, under these conditions blood would increase it's velocity at the distal side. Should this be the situation, then diffusion would be ineffective because the velocity of blood would be so fast that diffusion would not be possible.

Principle 3 defines that "...in the fluid transport system, the total cross sectional areas of the small vessels greatly exceeds that of large vessels, so flow velocities in the small vessels are lower than those in the large vessels". The arterial system transports blood under high pressure to tissues. The compliance of the arteries is such that a decrease in arterial blood pressure is directly proportional to the vascular resistance of that segment. In the aorta and large arteries this pressure loss is so minimal that a vessel 3 mm in diameter will have a pressure of about 95-97 mmHg. In the arteriole the resistance escalates rapidly, so that eventually almost half of the resistance of the vascular system occurs here. These vessels serve as control valves that regulate blood flow to the tissues. When blood enters the capillary system, it's pressure is usually about 30 mmHg . This is the exchange region where nutrients, waste products, electrolytes and other substances are exchanged between the intravascular and interstitial spaces. The pressure decrease across the short diffuse capillaries is about 20 mmHg. Therefore, as blood enters the venous system it does so against a pressure of about 10 mmHg. Blood is then collected by the venules and conducted back to the heart through the veins.

Principle 4 (Murray's Law) states that "....in an optimally designed system involving bulk laminar flow of an Newtonian fluid through pipes, at any branch point the radius of the parent vessel cubed will equal the sum of the cubes of the radii of the daughter vessels." According to Murray's Law, the flow disturbance at branch points is minimized as confirmed by flow visualization and pressure drop studies. As the radius of one vessel changes for whatever reason, change must be propagated at other junctions virtually throughout the system thus requiring a reorganization of the system. In order to substantiate Murray's Law, two observations need to be taken into account. Initially, the sheer stress on the walls of every vessel regardless of size must be the same. Secondly, the endothelial cells lining the vessels of the circulatory system should be sensitive to local sheer stress. Shear stress induces changes in the voltage across the cell membranes which alters the flow of ions through the cell membranes, resulting in a modification of proteins manufactured by these endothelial cells. When blood flow is altered as it may happen in surgical interventions or other situations, dramatic changes in shear stresses may occur. These changes are followed by alterations of vessel diameter in the surrounding tissues. The process occur within a few days and continue for months. Such remodeling can only happen when the involved vessels are lined with endothelial cells. Should the endothelial layer be removed or destroyed, then change in the flow of blood throughout the tissue can no longer accommodate change.[17-20]

VASCULAR SYSTEM CONTROL

The vascular system and the blood flow within, are controlled by various factors, such as the concentrations of metabolic nutrients, the concentrations of metabolic waste products, pressure receptors, and the autonomic nervous system.

When the concentration of oxygen in the tissue remain in normal range, there is little or no alteration in blood flow. However, should oxygen concentration in local tissue decrease, then the blood flow will concomitantly increase. As long as the adaptive changes can maintain the local tissue oxygenation, this new level of blood flow will be maintained. However, if the oxygen supply is insufficient, the precapillary sphincter muscle would have the tendency to relax. The relaxation occurs because oxygen is necessary for the contraction of the smooth muscle. When the oxygen concentration falls to anaerobic levels, the sphincter will open again, probably as a result of accumulation of vasodilator substances. The longer the vessel remains constricted and blood flow to the distal tissue continues to be compromised, the greater is the rate of formation of vasodilator mediators. These vasodilator substances are believed to diffuse back to the precapillary sphincters, and act as local regulators. Substances which can act in such a capacity are carbon dioxide, lactic acid, adenosine phosphate compounds, histamine, potassium and hydrogen.

When the blood supply to a tissue is blocked, and is followed by reperfusion, reactive hyperemia occurs. Reperfusion usually increases blood flow in the ischemic area to about 5 times normal. Generally, it continues for a few seconds or for as long as necessary in order to repay the oxygen debt created during the ischemic phase.

The autonomic nervous system plays an active role in the regulation of the heart function and circulatory system. The parasympathetic system exerts control over the heart's ability to function, and the sympathetic system innervates the vasculature. Sympathetic tone maintains the vessels in a state of partial constriction. The hypothalamus can exert excitatory or inhibitory effects which are then relayed to the sympathetic system which will elicit the desired action on the vessel. Vasoconstrictor substances such as norepinephrine act directly on the alpha- receptors located in all vessels except capillaries, precapillary sphincters and some arterioles, and act to change the capacitance of the affected vessel.

Under normal conditions the vasoconstrictor area transmits signals continuously through the sympathetic nerve fibers causing continuous slow firing and a partial state of contraction of the blood vessel. This normal situation becomes altered by extensive sympathetic stimulation or inhibition.[21] The arterial pressure is controlled by the baroreceptor reflexes. Any increase in arterial pressure which stretches the walls of the major arteries in the thorax and neck will excite these stretch receptors. Once stimulated, the signals are transmitted to the vasomotor center of the brain stem. The appropriate reflex signals are transmitted back to the heart and blood vessels. In the case of hypertension, bradycardia and vasodilatation occur. When an increased blood volume occurs, it is detected by the increased pressure in the central veins and the right and left atrium where stretch receptors are also located. Signals from the vasomotor center are then transmitted to the kidneys to increase urinary output.

OTHER VASOACTIVE SUBSTANCES

There are many vasoactive substances which are of interest to the perfusionist. An increase in Ca^{++} concentration causes vasoconstriction because it stimulates the smooth muscle. An increase in K^{+} concentration causes vasodilation because it's ability to inhibit smooth muscle contraction. Mg^{++}, a powerful vasodilator, is stimulated by an increase in ion concentration and inhibits smooth muscle contraction. Na^{+} concentration causes arteriolar dilatation. In addition, hyperglycemia can produce arteriolar dilatation by increasing blood osmolality. A decrease in blood osmolality can cause arteriolar constriction. An increase in the hydrogen ion concentration (low pH) causes dilatation of the arterioles, although a slight decrease in hydrogen ion concentration may cause arteriolar constriction. High levels of carbon dioxide cause moderate vasodilation in most tissues and marked dilatation in the brain.

THE EFFECTS OF CPB

Perfusion-induced alterations in physiology can have profound consequences. Aside from the induction of anesthesia which suppresses most of the regulatory mechanisms, and the impact of the surgical procedure, CPB induces anticoagulation, hemodilution, hypothermia and for the most part, pulseless blood flow. The changes induced by these perfusion techniques need to be identified.

During CPB most institutions serving the adult population utilize hemodilution to approximately 30% of total blood volume. This level of hemodilution causes changes in the blood rheology. The intention of hemodilution is to decrease the concentration of circulating blood elements. Thus, the fluid volume can be expanded to fill the artificially created enlarged perfusion vascular space without addition of homologous blood products.[22] The addition of acellular fluids causes other solutes to become diluted. The overall effect is a reduction in the concentration gradient needed for diffusion. The reduced gradient could possibly hinder the transfer of substrates and metabolites. One of the initial effects of hemodilution is a decrease in viscosity, and therefore, a reduction of those factors related to or dependent upon viscosity. The viscous effects of both blood compartments, cellular and plasma, will also be reduced by about 30%.[23] The additional viscous effects of the Fahreus-Linqvist factor will probably be enhanced because the counterforces will be minimized. A reduction in viscosity may facilitate tissue perfusion at the lower perfusion pressures found on bypass. The parabolic profile changes because less viscous friction is developed. This will allow the axial velocity to increase resulting in a longer parabola. The sheer stress and viscous friction between the vessel wall and formed elements, will also decrease because the diluent is less viscous than the original fluid. The ability of turbulent flow to result from laminar flow will be easier because the Reynold's number is inversely related to viscosity, and as the parabola becomes long it becomes more unstable, making the onset of turbulence easier. The heat release, resulting from the viscous friction will also significantly decline proportionally with the declining hematocrit and friction.

Reduced viscosity results in a decreased resistance to blood flow through the capillaries resulting in a enhanced tissue perfusion to a degree that might help compensate for the reduction in hematocrit. Blood velocity may improve in the capillaries with reduction of vascular resistance. The reduction in viscosity also allows for an increase in calculated blood flow rates to be achieved with lower perfusion pressures. Some studies have shown that hemodilution progressively increases cerebral blood flow,[24] and others state that as long as cerebral perfusion pressure can be maintained, the brain can tolerate a severe reduction in hemoglobin content.[25] Hemodilution may affect the buffering ability of the blood because of a reduction of the buffer contained within the hemoglobin[26]. Since it is hemoglobin dependent, the oxygen carrying capacity of the perfusion solution will also decrease. Additionally, the concentration of nutrients will also be reduced.

Another perfusion-related problem is *hypothermia*. Usually employed to a reduction of about 10 C^0 from normal, it has both metabolic and rheologic effects. Induced hypothermia will reduce the metabolic demands of the body in such a way that the nutrients needed for the maintenance of the body metabolism will be reduced in direct proportion to the reduction in temperature. Hypothermia reduces the need for oxygen, and exerts an effect on the rate of diffusion. As less oxygen and nutrients are needed and less waste is produced, the diffusion gradient becomes smaller with less demand on the intravascular resupply network. During hypothermia, the molecules will move less readily, resulting in an increase in viscosity. With a decrease in blood temperature, the oxyhemoglobin dissociation curve shifts to the left. Since the solubility of a gas in a liquid is inversely related to temperature, more oxygen is physically carried in the solution of the blood at the colder temperature. This probably maintains the status of the precapillary sphincter tone even in the presence of a reduced hematocrit. According to Bohr's effect, a decrease in temperature increases the carrying capacity of carbon dioxide and increases the activity of blood buffers. As blood is cooled, it is subjected to an increased solubility to carbon dioxide and a decreased dissociation and reduction of hydrogen ion activity. It has been reported that for each degree fall in temperature, oxygen consumption is reduced by 10%. The reduced need for oxygen implies that the metabolic rate decreases linearly at a temperature range between 22°C and 37°C. Hypothermia does not alter or reduce cerebral blood flow.[27] A detailed review of the subject of optimal perfusion flows was recently written by Mitchell.[23]

PULSELESS PERFUSION

The pulse pressure represents the difference between the systolic and diastolic pressure. In most centers, during routine CPB, the pulse pressures are either attenuated or nonexistent. These changes in pressures can cause immediate changes in blood flow in most tissue beds. As the arterial pressure becomes excessive, the increased flow provides excessive nutrients to the tissue and removes too much of the vasodilator mediators causing vasoconstriction, thus reducing local blood flow. Conversely, if the pressure and the blood flow drop to lower levels, an accumulation of vasodilatory substances will occur causing a further increase in vascular tone.

A correlation is reported by several studies between low mean arterial pressure and numerous neurological deficits.[28-30] Other studies have shown that the presence of neurological deficits relates inversely to blood flow rates. A pressure below 50 mmHg for protracted period, even at 20-30°C will result in severe neurological damage in the presence of pre-existing cerebral vascular disorders. An arterial pressure below 50 mmHg may be the critical level at which an electrocortical depression occurs and further decrease represents a significant contributor to cerebral ischemia. The association between the regional cerebral blood flow and mean arterial pressure is consistent with preserved autoregulation. Other investigators[31] have shown preservation of cerebral bloodflow with the presence of a pulse. During hypothermic, hemodiluted CPB, the lower pressure limit of autoregulation appears to be as low as 30 mmHg. This is in contrast to normotensive, normothermic individuals with normal cerebral vascular status in whom autoregulation maintains a constant cerebral blood flow between 50 mmHg and 150 mmHg pressure. Others have concluded that the lower limit of cerebral autoregulation is extended during hypothermic cardiopulmonary bypass at a pump output of 1.6 l/m^2. Another study shows a marked increase in flow during hyperemia. This flow gradually subsided but never returned to preload levels.[32] Under these conditions, pharmacological support is not deemed necessary to maintain cerebral blood flow between a mean arterial pressure of 30 mmHg-110 mmHg. A direct relationship between hematocrit and viscosity is apparently cancelled by hypothermia because whole blood has a 5% increase in viscosity with each Celsius degree drop in temperature.

Nonpulsatile perfusion means the absence of a distal pulse pressure. The normal stretching and relaxation of the arterial system is replaced by a steady flow and pressure. This may be detrimental to the microcirculation. Under these conditions, it may be inaccurate to use Reynold's number to calculate turbulence for pulsatile blood flow.[33]

The normal compliance of the aorta may be eliminated with pulseless perfusion because peripheral vascular resistance increases with comparable flow rates. Since there is no diastolic time to allow the aorta to unload (constrict), it appears that once the aorta is filled it's compliance will continue to decrease. A comparison of mean pressures indicates that a higher flow rate is required with pulsatile perfusion in order to maintain comparable pressures. If comparable mean pressures are maintained by increasing flow, pulsatile perfusion leads to improve aerobic systemic metabolism which is associated with measurable increases in systemic oxygen consumption and lower lactate levels. Renal perfusion has been shown to be improved by pulsatile flow.[34] The lack of a pulse pressure over time has significant ramifications on the ability of the body to effectively metabolize. Diffusion is impaired. In order for the diffusive process to work, the capillaries need the energy present in the pulsatile wave in order to maintain capillary integrity and pressure differential. In the case of a loss or lack of pulsatile flow, high blood flows would have to be established in the aorta from the perfusion pump. These steady state flows may create turbulence because of the high rate at which blood should be pumped in order to meet metabolic demands. As previously described, turbulent blood becomes ineffective in the delivery process of nutrients to the periphery.

CONCLUSION

Vogel[35] defines a circulatory system as "...devices that use some form of convective bulk flow to reduce the effective distance between two parts of an organism or between the organism and it's environment." The perfusion circulatory system fulfills these criteria and goes a step further in that it connects the living organism with an artificially constructed environment. Currently, many unexplained phenomena result from the patient's interaction with this artificial environment. Probably the most interesting observation is that, there is an extremely high number of patients undergoing CPB with little or no sequalae at all.

REFERENCES

1. M. LaBarbera: Inner Currents, How fluid dynamics channels natural selection. *The Sciences* 30:37;1991.
2. T.C. Hung, D.B. Butter, R.L. Kormos, et al: Characteristics of blood rheology in patients during Novacor left ventricular assist system support. *ASAIO Trans* 35(3):611-3;1989.
3. G. de Simone, R.B. Devereux, S.Chien, M.H. Alderman, S.A. Atlas, J.H. Laragh: Relation of blood viscosity to demographic and physiologic variables and to cardiovascular risk factors in apparently normal adults. *Circulation* 81(1):107-117;1990.

4. M.M. Guest, T.P. Bond, R.G. Cooper, J.R. Derrick: Red blood cells: change in shape in capillaries. *Science* 142:1319-1321;1963.
5. G.T. DePalma: Hemodynamics of arterial blood flow. In: *The Basic Science of Vascular Surgery*, edited by Giordano JM, Trout HH, DePalma RG, Futura, Mount Kisco, p 113;1988.
6. L. Hatle, B. Angelsen: Physics of blood flow: physical principles and clinical applications. In: *Doppler Ultrasound in Cardiology*. Second Edition. Lea & Febiger, Philadelphia, 1982.
7. C.C. Reed, T.B. Stafford: Flow-Pressure-Resistance. In: *Cardiopulmonary Bypass* Second Edition, p 157;1985.
8. M. Nelkin: In what sense is turbulence an unsolved problem? *Science* 255:566-570;1992.
9. L. Hatle, B. Angelsen: Physics of blood flow. In: *Doppler Ultrasound in Cardiology* Third Edition, Lea & Febiger, Philadelphia, p 81;1988.
10. S. Vogel: How blood moves in pumps, pipes, and the workings of circulatory systems. *Vital Circuits*, Oxford Univ Press, New York 81;1992.
11. M. Motomiya, Karino T: Flow patterns in the human carotid artery bifurcation. *Stroke* 15:50-56;1984.
12. A.C. Guyton: *Textbook of Medical Physiology*: Seventh Edition W.B. Saunders Co, Philadelphia, p 211;1986.
13. A.C. Guyton, *Textbook of Medical Physiology*: Seventh Edition W.B. Saunders Co, Philadelphia, p 227;1986.
14. A.P. Shepherd, G.L. Riedel: Effect of pulsatile pressure and metabolic rate on intestinal autoregulation. *Am J Physiol* 242:H769-H775;1982.
15. R.F. Rushmer: Functional anatomy and control of the heart. In: *Cardiovascular Dynamics*, Edited by R.F. Rushmer, Fourth Edition, W.B. Saunders Co., Philadelphia, p 97;1988.
16. M. LaBarbera: Principles of design of fluid transport systems in zoology. *Science* 249:992-1000;1990.
17. K. Perktold, M. Resch: Numerical flow studies in human carotid artery bifurcations: Basic discussion of the geometric factor in atherogenesis. *J Biomed Eng* 12:111-23;1990.
18. T. Asakura, T. Karino: Flow patterns and spatial distribution of atherosclerotic lesions in human coronary arteries. *Circulation Research* 66:1045-1066;1990.
19. C.K. Zarins, D.P. Giddens, B.K. Bharadvaj, V.S. Sottiurai, R. F. Mabon, S. Glagov: Carotid bifurcation atherosclerosis: quantitative correlation of plaque localization with flow velocity profiles and wall shear stress. *Circ Research* 53:502-14;1983.
20. M.J. Levesque, D. Liepsch, S. Moravec, R.M. Nerem: Correlation of endothelial cell shape and wall shear stress in a stenosed dog aorta. *Arteriosclerosis* 6:220-229;1986.
21. C.J. Jones: Autonomic nerves and the control of blood flow: Theory and Practice. In: *Blood Flow - Theory and Practice*, 16:272.
22. F. Gollan: Carbon dioxide, waste product, or elixir? *J Mount Sinai Hosp* 32:132;1965.
23. B.A. Mitchell: Optimal perfusion flow rates for cardiopulmonary bypass. *J Extra-Corp Tech* 22:165-183;1991.
24. I.R. Thomson: The influence of cardiopulmonary bypass on cerebral physiology and function. In: *Cardiopulmonary Bypass: Current Concepts and Controversies*, Edited by J.H. Tinker, W.B. Saunders Co., Philadelphia, p 21-40;1989.
25. P. Bard: *Medical Physiology*, 10th Edition, Mosby Co., St. Louis, 1956.
26. E.G.Brewin: Physiology of hypothermia. *Int Anesth Clin* 2:803-826;1964.

27. A.Okuda, et al: Experimental studies on the relationship between whole body oxygen consumption and perfusion flow rate. *J Jpn Assoc Thorac Surg* 31:1057-1069;1983.
28. H. Javid, H.M. Tufo, H. Najafi, et al: Neurologic abnormalities following open-heart surgery. *J Thorac Cardiovasc Surg* 58:502-9;1969.
29. I. Juneja, R.E. Flynn, R.L. Berger: The arterial and venous pressure and the electroencephalogram during open-heart surgery. *Acta Neuro Scand* 48:163-8;1971.
30. J.A.V. Govier, J.G. Reves, R.D. McKay, et al: Factors and their influence on regional cerebral blood flow during nonpulsatile cardiopulmonary bypass. *Ann Thorac Surgery* 38:592-600;1984.
31. G.A. Taylor, G.R. Martin, B.L. Short: Cardiac determinants of cerebral blood flow during extracorporeal membrane oxygenation. *Invest Radiol* 24:511-516;1989.
32. R.A. Frantz, G.C. Xakellis: Characteristics of skin blood flow over the trochanter under constant, prolonged pressure. *Am J Phys Med Rehab* 68:272-6;1989.
33. D.N. Ku, D.P. Giddens, C.K. Zarins, S. Glagov: Pulsatile flow and atherosclerosis in the human carotid bifurcation - Positive correlation between plaque location and low and oscillating shear stress. *Arteriosclerosis* 5:293-302;1985.
34. K. Nakayama, T. Tamiya, K. Yamamoto, et al: High amplitude pulsatile pump in extracorporeal circulation with particular reference to hemodynamics. *Surgery* 54:798;1963.
35. S. Vogel: Why move blood? In: *Vital Circuits*. Edited by S. Vogel, Oxford Univ Press, New York, 6:105;1992.

POSTOPERATIVE RESPONSES TO HYPOTHERMIA: NURSING CONSIDERATIONS

Jill A. Fikkert, BSN, R.N.

Visiting Nurses of South Central Connecticut
New Haven, Connecticut

Recognition of hypothermia in the postoperative cardiac surgery patient by the critical care nurse is essential to safe and prudent nursing management of this patient population. Admitting nurses naturally focus on the immediate tasks of attaching EKG leads and arterial lines to the monitor, titrating vasopressors, placing the chest tubes to suction, and connecting foley catheters to straight drainage; all the while their patient is at risk for further hypothermia due to the fact that by the time the patient is transported to the intensive care unit, core temperatures can fall to hypothermic levels again.[1] Keeping the patient warm may seem less vital than controlling hypertension and bleeding; however, by taking a few preventive measures to avert further hypothermia and to promote active rewarming nurses can significantly improve patients' postoperative recovery phase. Nurses play a key role in prompt assessment, immediate response, and appropriate intervention. The remainder of this chapter discusses the clinical levels of hypothermia, the clinical uses of hypothermia during cardiopulmonary bypass, the physiologic effects of hypothermia on body systems, the intrinsic and extrinsic methods of rewarming, and pharmacologic support and nursing interventions.

CLINICAL LEVELS OF HYPOTHERMIA

Prior to an understanding of the effects of hypothermia on the cardiac surgery patient, it is imperative that the practitioner have an adequate awareness of the clinical levels of hypothermia. Normothermia includes a temperature range of 36.6-37.5°C or 97.9-99.5°F. At these temperatures enzyme function that is responsible for acid/base

Cardiac Surgery: Current Issues, Edited by A.C. Cernaianu and A.J. DelRossi Plenum Press, New York, 1992

balance and clotting mechanisms are stabilized.[2,3] Mild hypothermia is defined as 34.0-36.5°C or 93.2-97.0°F, which is the temperature range at which the patient returns from the operating room. Unfortunately, it has been found that the exposure of the patient's skin during transport tends to drop body temperatures 1-2°C.[1] Unlike mild hypothermia, moderate hypothermia is experienced by the patient in the operating room. The temperature ranges are 28.0-33.5°C or 82.4-92.3°F. Notably, it has been found that at this temperature range ventricular fibrillation is easily precipitated. The last two clinical levels of hypothermia are deep hypothermia (17.0-27.5°C or 62.6-81.5°F) and profound hypothermia (4.0-16.5°C or 39.2-61.7°F), both of which have no clinical significance for the cardiac surgery population.

CLINICAL USE OF HYPOTHERMIA DURING CARDIOPULMONARY BYPASS

The basis for the use of cooling in the cardiopulmonary bypass arises from the fact that it decreases the metabolic rate, thereby decreasing oxygen demands. The metabolic and oxygen demands of tissues are reduced during circulatory diversion when the body temperature is lowered below 30°C (moderate hypothermia). It has been noted that with each 10°C drop in body temperature there is a decline of about 7-10 percent in metabolic demands.[4] Systemic hypothermia in conjunction with cold chemical cardioplegia continues to be the standard technique for myocardial preservation during open heart surgery. The cardioplegic solution is reinfused into the aortic root every 20-30 minutes or when myocardial activity resumes. The cardioplegia solutions are 4°C when they are infused into the aortic root.[5] Cardiopulmonary bypass is not without adverse effects. For example, blood viscosity rises when the body temperature is lowered and may result in sluggish capillary and organ blood flow.

NEUROLOGICAL EFFECTS OF HYPOTHERMIA

According to Feldman, cerebral blood flow decreases by 6-7 percent for every 1°C drop in temperature.[6] Diminished cerebral blood flow results in a desensitizing of the sensorium and of the thought processes. The central nervous system is further depressed as the temperature continues to drop. There is a decreased metabolic need for oxygen and glucose by the brain in the hypothermic syndrome which is a protective mechanism against the loss of cerebral blood flow.[6] It is because of this desensitized sensorium that it is crucial for the nurse to assess the patient's level of orientation while awakening from anesthesia postoperatively. It is imperative that the patient is oriented to the environment. It is likely that nurses may overlook this mental sluggishness since the disorientation resolves as the patient moves towards normothermia and recovers from anesthesia. Immediately upon the termination of anesthesia, shivering begins in response to the demand for heat generation as the thermoregulatory center resumes functioning. Shivering as a means of heat production is known to increase postoperative oxygen consumption to over 400 percent of basal oxygen requirements.[7] The postoperative oxygen consumption in the shivering patient places a substantial burden on the cardio-pulmonary system, raising the patent's heart rate and blood pressure. This obviously has a deleterious effect on the cardiac surgery patient.

CARDIOVASCULAR EFFECTS OF HYPOTHERMIA

The cardiovascular effects of hypothermia are among the most serious in terms of the consequences that they present to the cardiac surgery patient. Vasoconstriction reflects the body's effort to conserve heat in response to cold. Feroe and Augustine note that the constriction of the arterioles results in hypertension, which can lead to excessive bleeding from the chest tubes and also to pressure on the newly-bypassed vessel.[8] A secondary effect of vasoconstriction is an increase in cardiac workload because the heart is pumping against a greater pressure gradient, adding stress to the recovering heart. A tertiary side effect is tachycardia, which is a compensatory response to facilitate additional cardiac output. Tachycardia poses the most serious threat to the patient with coronary artery disease.[8] The patient experiences regional vasoconstriction from the release of catecholamines as a result of the surgery. Numerous factors predispose the cardiac surgery patient to significant elevations in systemic vascular resistance. Some of these factors are: the effects of cardiopulmonary bypass, pain, agitation, shivering, hypoxia, hypercarbia, and withdrawal of antihypertensive medications. Such increases in afterload can critically intensify myocardial oxygen demands and significantly reduce cardiac output. An elevated systemic vascular resistance can mask significant hypovolemia in these patients as they are warmed and vasodilate in the postoperative period. Other significant cardiovascular effects of hypothermia are conduction disturbances and arrhythmias. Both are caused by the irritation of the myocardium in the hypothermic syndrome, by alterations in acid/base balance, by inadequate tissue oxygenation, and by the effects of cold on the heart. The most prevalent EKG abnormalities are T wave inversions, interval prolongations, and the J wave, the latter considered to be the classic diagnostic sign of hypothermia. One of the arrhythmias commonly seen is sinus bradycardia, so it is important to have a functioning pacemaker in order that the patient can be temporarily paced should this occur. A second arrhythmia is atrial fibrillation, which frequently develops at temperatures less than 32.3°C as a result of atrial distension. Premature ventricular contractions are also common and if not corrected can deteriorate into ventricular fibrillation, which often happens at temperatures less than 28 C.[6,9] It is imperative that EKG abnormalities and conduction disturbances be accurately and swiftly identified and expeditiously corrected in order to restore cardiovascular stability.

PULMONARY EFFECTS OF HYPOTHERMIA

Associated with a decrease in oxygen uptake is a decrease in carbon dioxide production and an increase in solubility of carbon dioxide leading to a decrease in the respiratory quotient. Acidosis may be caused by carbon dioxide retention due to respiratory failure or tissue hypoxia and metabolic acidosis and microcirculatory failure.[10] A second pulmonary effect of hypothermia is an increase in oxygen consumption due to shivering to a level of 2-5 times the resting rate.[11] Hypothermia has an effect on the oxyhemoglobin disassociation curve, shifting it to the left and thus increasing the affinity for oxygen. When oxygen becomes more tightly bound to the hemoglobin it is less available for use to the tissues; however, Reuler states that this is not usually clinically significant because of the concomitant decrease in oxygen requirement.[10] Increasing the concentration or rate of oxygen administration to the patient with increased requirements (i.e. shivering) will not meet the higher demand in every instance. In addition, the patient's respiratory rate and tidal volume are initially increased, but as the basal metabolic rate is lowered the respiratory rate and tidal volume decrease.

GASTROINTESTINAL EFFECTS OF HYPOTHERMIA

Intestinal motility decreases below 34°C and ileus is a commonly observed phenomenon.[4] This is why it is shared practice to insert nasogastric tubes prior to the onset of the surgery. An ileus may be easily diagnosed by viewing the postoperative x-ray. Should this phenomenon occur, the abdomen should be regularly assessed for bowel sounds and all oral intake held until this is resolved. Moreover, hypothermia inhibits the release of insulin from the pancreas as well as the peripheral use of glucose, causing hyperglycemia. These abnormalities, however, revert with rewarming and therefore the use of insulin to correct hyperglycemia may run the risk of hypoglycemia. Shivering may also deplete glycogen stores and further aggravate hypoglycemia.[12] The detoxification and conjugation activities of the liver are also depressed, causing drugs to remain in the system for prolonged periods of time with obvious multiple untoward effects.[4]

RENAL EFFECTS OF HYPOTHERMIA

Urine output should be assessed by the nurse to evaluate the effectiveness of the patient's cardiac output and for the possibility of acute tubular necrosis. Acute tubular necrosis rarely occurs because of the improved cardiopulmonary bypass techniques, however, it is still a possibility.[13] Urine flow increases with decreased temperatures (cold diuresis) secondary to depressed oxidative tubular activity, which results in reduced sodium and water resorption. This combined with shifts of fluids to the extracellular space may render the patient hypovolemic.[14,15] It is important to assess the patient for hypovolemia because of the vulnerability to hypovolemia from several sources.

HEMATOLOGIC EFFECTS OF HYPOTHERMIA

The hematologic effects of hypothermia include an elevated hematocrit and a depressed leucocyte and platelet count. The hematocrit is elevated secondary to plasma loss and splenic contraction with an increase in viscosity at temperatures less than 27°C.[16]

Leucocyte and platelet counts are commonly depressed secondary to splenic, hepatic, and intravascular sequestration. Disseminated intravascular coagulation has been a feature in some cases.[17,18]

NURSING IMPLICATIONS OF REWARMING

The nursing implications of rewarming are twofold, involving both intrinsic and extrinsic methods for thermoregulation. The central nervous system responds to changes in temperature gradients between thermoreceptors and the internal and/or external environment.[19] The intrinsic mechanisms for thermoregulation consist of the release of endogenous catecholamines and stimulation of the posterior hypothalamus. The release of endogenous catecholamines leads to vasoconstriction. The autonomic nervous system indirectly influences shivering by release of catecholamines, heightening muscle tone and prompting vasoconstriction which leads to further tissue cooling. Cold blood from the periphery is returned suddenly to the central circulation which results in a decrease in core temperature and myocardial irritability.[20]

A second intrinsic mechanism is the stimulation of the posterior hypothalamus which leads to shivering. This usually occurs within the first four post-operative hours, a time of high staff activity which may cause the shivering to go unnoticed by the primary caregiver.[19] There are several ways for the professional nurse to detect shivering. The first is through arterial blood gas interpretation. There is a decrease in arterial and venous oxygen saturation and a falling pH.[19] In the past it was also possible to detect shivering secondary to the artifact in the EKG tracing; however, with the advent of more sophisticated technology, EKGs are now designed to filter out the artifact. Nevertheless, if the patient's shivering is sufficiently profound, the artifact can still be easily seen on the EKG tracing. Finally, shivering may be detected through what is termed a mandibular vibration or hum. In order to determine this occurrence it is necessary to place the fingers along the edges of the patient's jaw. According to Holtzclaw, this occurs prior to visible shivering.[19] While it is helpful for the nurse to recognize the intrinsic mechanisms for thermoregulation, it is equally imperative for the nurse to be knowledgeable regarding the various methods for extrinsic regulation. The first and most basic method is a warm environment. While operating rooms are generally kept at temperatures less than 21°C, intensive care units are wisely kept warmer.

Cotton blankets are a second means to rewarm the hypothermic patient. Reuler was the first to recognize that cotton blankets offer only the benefits of passive rewarming because of the low specific heat.[10] Cotton blanket therapy fails to meet the primary objective in the treatment of the hypothermic patient: cotton blankets do not actively heat the patient.[8] Despite their apparent passive effects, blankets are often the only means to begin the process of rewarming. Cotton blankets are more effective if they are warmed via a blanket warmer. It is not wise to warm blankets in a microwave due to the potential for fire. It is also imperative for the nurse to be alert to the possibility for burns secondary to decreased circulation as well as the added danger of burns related to betadine on the skin coming into contact with the heat.

Fluid circulating blankets are a third and controversial way of rewarming the patient post-operatively. Fluid circulating blankets are known to burn, again in connection with betadine. These blankets are also known to rewarm too rapidly, creating a stressor for the already compromised cardiovascular system by rapidly increasing the metabolic rate and consumption of oxygen.

Rewarming encourages acidosis by causing constricted peripheral vascular beds to open and load the circulation with fixed acids and metabolites.[8] Head coverings are a safe, easy, inexpensive, and effective means of preventing further heat loss. This is a solution which can be implemented intra-operatively and be continued postoperatively as well. A person's head is responsible for as much as 50 percent of the body's total heat loss. This heat loss results from the shunting of circulating blood volume to the head during extremes in thermal gradients.[21]

An additional aid to rewarming is radiant lighting, which involves warming the environment directly surrounding the patient. Published evidence suggests that radiant lighting does not actively rewarm adults.[22-25] The reasons for this ineffectiveness are that direct exposure of the skin is required for radiant lighting and that only a small area at the body's center perpendicular to the heat source maximally absorbs heat. It is important to remember that it is next to impossible to leave a patient exposed in a busy intensive care unit, not to mention the fact that such exposure leaves the patient open to further decreases in temperatures. When using radiant lighting, the lights should be turned off when the patient's temperature reaches 97-98°F in order that the patient does not become hyperthermic.

Inhalation of warm, humidified air via the endotracheal tube is also used to prevent heat loss. Tausk et al found that humidifying the patient's gases during prolonged anesthesia decreases lung damage and prevents the development of hypothermia.[26]

The newest technology in temperature regulation is known as convective warming therapy, a technique which transfers heat to the patient by blowing warm air through a plastic and tissue paper blanket that covers the patient. Microperforations on the underside of the blanket direct warm air-streams onto the patient's skin. Even at the lowest temperature setting, convective warming therapy was proven to be more effective than the warm-water blankets or radiant lighting.[27]

PHARMACOLOGIC SUPPORT AND NURSING INTERVENTIONS

Drugs may be given to suppress shivering by eradicating the hypothalamic response to stimuli through depressing spinal reflexes or by interfering with the transmission of neuromuscular impulses.[19] Vasodilators are the first category of drugs used to aid in rewarming. Nipride has been used to rewarm the patient more evenly.[28,29] By avoiding vasoconstriction during rewarming, temperature rises gradually and more uniformly without the rapid shifts and steep gradients that promote shivering. It is useful for vasodilator drugs to be combined with the use of blankets to help prevent heat loss due to the patient's lack of ability to conserve heat. It is important to remember that peripheral resistance is lowered, so it is necessary to monitor fluid and hemodynamic status closely to avoid hypovolemia.[19]

Narcotics and benzodiazapines are a second form of pharmacologic support. Narcotics such as morphine and demerol are used successfully after surgery to suppress shivering.[30] It has been found that a patient receiving narcotics in doses sufficient to stop shivering will have a prolonged rewarming period. Valium and Versed are often used in conjunction with morphine and neuromuscular blocking agents. Versed has often been found to be a wiser choice in consideration of the patient's respiratory status. Versed has a shorter half-life than valium and is 3-4 times more potent. Because of its shorter half-life, extubation may be performed more quickly.

Finally, neuromuscular blockade is one of the most successful methods of shivering control. Metocurine iodine is used to suppress shivering during passive rewarming and has been found to improve hemodynamic and cardiorespiratory stability.[31] Pavulon is also commonly used, but it has been found to have reflex tachycardia and to increase arterial blood pressures. Remember when using neuromuscular blockade to suppress shivering, it is important to use an additional drug such as morphine or valium.

REFERENCES

1. B. Holtzclaw: Temperature problems in the postoperative period. *Critical Care Nursing Clinics of North America* 2:589-597;1990.
2. F.A. White: A comparative physiological approach to hypothermia. *J Thor Cardiovasc Surg* 82:821-831;1981.
3. R. Eberhart, A. Shitaer (Eds.): *Heat transfer in medicine and biology, analysis and applications* vol 1 New York, Plenum Press;1985.
4. E. Blair: *Clinical Hypothermia* New York, McGraw Hill, 19-22;1964.
5. K. Litwack, F. Hicks, D. Brooks: Practical points in the care of the patient postcardiac surgery. *J Post Anesthesia Nursing* 5:106-111;1990.
6. L.D. Vandam, T.K. Burnap: Hypothermia. *N Engl J Med* 261:546-553;1959.
7. M.S. Vaughan, R.W. Vaughan, R.C. Cork: Postoperative hypothermia in adults: Relationship of age, anesthesia, and shivering to rewarming. *Anesth Analg* 60:746-751;1981.
8. D. Feroe, S. Augustine: Hypothermia in the PACU. *Critical Care Nursing Clinics of North America* 3:135-144;1991.
9. C.V. Mouritzen, M.N. Andersen: Myocardial temperature gradients and ventricular fibrillation during hypothermia. *J Thor Cardiovasc Surg* 49:937-944;1965.
10. J. Reuler: Hypothermia, pathophysiology, clinical settings, and management. *Ann Int Med* 89:519-527;1989.
11. A. Hemingway: Shivering. *Physiology Review* 43:401;1963.
12. D.L. Curry, K.P. Curry: Hypothermia and insulin secretion. *Endocrinology* 87:750-755;1970.
13. B.M. Hightower, M.R. Kinney: Extracorporeal circulation. *AACN's Clinical Reference for Critical Care Nursing* Edited by M.R. Kinney, McGraw-Hill, NY, p 949-955;1981.
14. J.H. Moyer, G. Morris, M.E. DeBakey: Hypothermia: effect on renal hypodynamics and on excretion of water and electrolytes in dog and man. *Ann Surgery* 145:26-40;1957.
15. W.E. Segar, P.A. Riley, T.G. Barila: Urinary composition during hypothermia. *Am J Physiol* 185:528-532;1956.
16. G.S. Kanter: Hypothermic hemoconcentration. *Am J Physiol* 214:856-859;1968.
17. M.A. Chad, O.P. Gray: Hypothermia and coagulation defects in the newborn. *Arch Dis Child* 47:819-821;1972.
18. J.T. Willson, W.R. Miller, T.S. Elliot: Blood studies in the hypothermic dog. *Surgery* 43:979-989;1958.
19. B. Holtzclaw: Postoperative shivering following cardiac surgery: A review. *Heart and Lung* 15(3):292-302;1986.
20. C. Biddle: Hypothermia: Implications for the critical care nurse. *Critical Care Nurse* 5(2):34-38;1985.
21. M. Blansett: The effects of rewarming hypothermic post anesthesia patients using thermadrape covering, heat lamps, and warmed cotton blankets. *J Post Anesth Nurs* 5:80-84;1990.
22. S. Hennenberg, A. Eklund, P.O. Joachimsson, et al: Effects of a thermal ceiling on postoperative hypothermia. *Acta Anesthesiol Scand* 29:602-606; 1985.
23. D.H. Kucha, G.A. Nichols, N.M. Christ, et al: The warming of postoperative patients. *Milit Med* 139:388-390;1974.
24. A. Sharkey, J.M. Lipton, M.T. Murphy, et al: Inhibition of postanesthetic shivering with radiant heat. *Anesthesiology* 66:249-252;1987.
25. M.S. Vaughn: Shivering in the recovery room. *Curr Rev RR Nurse* 6:2-7;1984.
26. H.C. Tausk, R. Miller, R.B. Roberts: Maintenance of body temperature by heated humidification. *Anesth Analg* 55:719-723;1976.

27. D.I. Sessler, A. Moayeri: Skin surface warming: Heat flux and central temperature. *Anesthesiology* 73:218-224;1990.
28. C.R. Noback, J.H. Tinker: Hypothermia after cardiopulmonary bypass in man: amelioration by nitroprusside-induced vasodilation during rewarming. *Anesthesiology* 53:277;1980.
29. K.G. Bridges, G.A. Reichard, H. Macvaugh, J.R. Kues, W.G. Cevallos, M.J. Lechman, W.S. Hoffman, J.S. Donahoo: Effect of phentolamine in controlling temperature and acidosis associated with cardiopulmonary bypass. *Crit Care Med* 13:72;1985.
30. J.L. Rodriguez, C. Weissman, M.C. Damask, J. Askanazi, A.I. Hyman, J.M. Kinney: Physiologic requirements during rewarming: suppression of the shivering response. *Crit Care Med* 11:496;1983.
31. J.L. Rodriguez, C. Weissman, M.C. Damask, J. Askanazi, A.I. Hyman, J.M.Kinney: Morphine and postoperative rewarming in critically ill patients. *Circulation* 68:1242;1983.
32. O. Chiara, P. Giomarelli, B. Biagiloi, R. Rosi, L. Gattiononi:Hypermetabolic response after hypothermic cardiopulmonary bypass. *Crit Care Med* 15:995-999;1987.
33. J.W. Dundee, R. King: Clinical aspects of induced hypothermia: Methods of production and indications for its use. *Br J Anaest* 31:106-133;1959.
34. M.D. Fallacaro, N.A. Fallacaro, L.T.J. Radel: Inadvertent hypothermia, etiology, effects, and prevention. *AORN J* 44:54-60;1986.
35. M.E. Feldman: Inadvertent hypothermia: a threat to homeostasis in the postanesthetic patient. *J Post Anesth Nurs* 3:82-87;1988.
36. K.E. Fraulini: Nursing Care of the postanesthetic patient, postanesthetic problems after anesthesia. *A Guide for PACU, ICU, and Medical-Surgical Nurses*. Norwalk, CT, Appleton and Lange, pp. 142-209;1987.
37. R. Ilia, I Ovsyschcher, L Rudnik, M Gueron: Atypical ventricular tachycardia and alternating osborn waves induced by spontaneous mild hypothermia. *Ped Cardiol* 9:63-65;1988.
38. S. Oliver, E. Fuessel: Control of postoperative hypothermia in cardiovascular surgery patients. *Critical Care Nurse Quarterly* 12:63-68;1990.
39. R. Phillips, P. Skov: Rewarming and cardiac surgery: a review. *Heart and Lung* 17(5):511-520;1988.
40. J. Slotman, H. Jed, W. Burchard: Adverse effects of hypothermia in postoperative patients. *Am J Surg* 149:495-500;1985.
41. S. Soukup: Accidental hypothermia. In M. Kinney, C. Dear, D. Packa, K. Voorman (Eds.): *AACN's Clinical Reference for Critical Care Nursing*. New York, Mcgraw-Hill, p 991-996;1981.
42. L. Villamiel: Help! this postanesthesia care unit patient is hypothermic. *Journal of Post Anesthesia Nursing* 5(2):75-79;1990.
43. J. Zwischenberger, M. Kirsch, R. Dechert, D. Arnold, R. Bartlett: Suppression of shivering decreases oxygen consumption and improves hemodynamic stability during postoperative rewarming. *Ann Thor Surg* 43:979-989;1987.

CARDIAC VALVE REPLACEMENT IN THE 1990s:

THE NURSING PERSPECTIVE

Susan Kiley Eckert, MSN, R.N., CCRN

Washington Hospital Center
Washington, DC

The cardiac surgical population, particularly those undergoing coronary artery bypass surgery (CABG) has changed significantly in the past decade. The explosion of interventional cardiology techniques and procedures has, in some cases, redefined the type of patient we see in the operating room, and Intermediate ICU, (stepdown units). Heart valve replacement and more recently valve repair, however, remains a compelling reason for undergoing open heart surgery. As in all other areas of health care, considerable research and development is taking place to improve the options and enhance patient outcomes. This chapter will review concepts and issues surrounding cardiac valve disease, surgical interventions to correct pathology and key nursing issues in managing patients post cardiac valve replacement/repair.

ETIOLOGIES OF VALVE DISEASE

Rheumatic fever remains a primary cause of acquired valvular heart disease - particularly mitral valves. However, there has been a decline in the incidence of rheumatic fever in the United States due to improved antibiotic therapy, changing virulence of group A streptococci and overall improvements in the health care delivery system that have led to increased access to health care for patients. Other problems however, may lead to the need for valve replacement or repair. Table 1 summarizes the common etiologies of valve disease. Knowledge of the cause of valve dysfunction is helpful in anticipating the consequences of the disease process. For instance, an acute event such as mitral regurgitation secondary to a traumatic event (i.e. shearing forces rupturing papillary muscle or chordae tendineae) may lead to immedi-

Cardiac Surgery: Current Issues, Edited by A.C. Cernaianu
and A.J. DelRossi Plenum Press, New York, 1992

TABLE 1. Etiologies of Valve Disease.

Mitral Stenosis	Mitral Regurgitation
Rheumatic Heart Disease	Rheumatic Heart Disease
Tumors	Endocarditis
Calcification	Prolapse
Vegetation	Trauma
Prothesis Dysfunction	Calcification
Aortic Stenosis	**Aortic Regurgitation**
Rheumatic Heart Disease	Rheumatic Heart Disease
Calcification	Trauma
	Arthritic Disease
	Syphilis
	Calcification
	Endocarditis
	Arteriosclerosis
	Aortic Aneurysm
	Hypertension

ate valve replacement. Heart muscle in this case would not have undergone the pathologic changes that typically occur as a result of a more chronic process - i.e. rheumatic heart disease. Nursing interventions, therefore would be refined to accommodate a relatively "healthy" heart in contrast to an organ that has sustained years of chronic changes.

VALVULAR PATHOLOGY: STENOSIS VS. REGURGITATION

Two primary pathologies are caused by valve dysfunction: stenosis & regurgitation. Regurgitation may also be known as insufficiency or incompetence. Stenosis is defined as a narrowing of the opening or orifice of the valve opening. A normal mitral valve orifice is 5-13 cm^2 with critical mitral stenosis occurring at 2.5 cm^2 or less, while a normal aortic valve orifice is 2.5-3.5 cm^2, with critical stenosis occurring at 0.6 cm^2 or less (adults). Regurgitation is defined as the incomplete closure of the valve orifice with subsequent systolic regurgitation of blood into the preceding chamber. The amount of insufficiency depends upon the severity and degree of resistance through the outflow tract. The identification of which type of pathology that led to the need for valve replacement or repair is crucial in determining postoperative management of the patient, as the pathology leads to unique changes in the heart muscle. Simplistically, stenosis typically leads to a hypertrophied ventricle while regurgitation leads to a dilated ventricle. These changes refine nursing management in the acute postoperative phase of recovery and will be discussed in more detail in that section. Tables 2 and 3 outline the potential physiologic consequences of mitral or aortic stenosis and regurgitation.

TABLE 2. Physiologic Consequences of Mitral Valve Disease.

Mitral stenosis		Mitral regurgitation	
↑ LA pressure	↓ CO	↑ LA Pressure	↓ C.O.
↓		↓	
LA hypertrophy		↑ PVR	
↓		↓	
Atrial Fibrillation	↑ PVR	↑ RV Pressure	
	↓	↓	
	↑ RV Pressure	RV dilatation/failure	
	↓	↓	
	RV hypertrophy	↑ RA pressure/CVP	
	↓		
	RV failure		

TABLE 3. Physiologic Consequences of Aortic Valve Disease.

Aortic stenosis		Aortic Regurgitation	
↓		↓	
LV hypertrophy		LV dilatation	
LV failure	LA hypertrophy	LV failure	LA dilatation
↓		↓	
↑ LA pressure		↑ LA pressure	
↓		↓	
↑ PVR		↑ PVR	
↓		↓	
↑ RV pressure		↑ RV pressure	
↓		↓	
↑ RA pressure/CVP		↑ RA	

MORTALITY/MORBIDITY

The overall mortality rate for patients undergoing cardiac valvular surgery is approximately 4-7%. Numerous studies have been published analyzing the efficacy of valve replacement vs. medical management, however, it is difficult to make too many generalizations due to the number of prosthesis on the market and the impact of patient variables on such data (i.e., age, preoperative status, surgical technique, etc.) Some inferences can be made regarding variables that favorably impact a patient's potential mortality.(Table 4) Patients who have exhibited cardiac symptoms for less than three years, those who fall in the New York Heart Association (NYHA) Functional classes 1 and 2, have had no previous myocardial infarctions (MI), and exhibit good left ventricular function and do not experience systemic or chronic illness (i.e. AODM, PVD, COPD, etc.) have a better chance for successfully undergoing cardiac valvular surgery. In addition, age of less than 60 years, valve dysfunction caused by rheumatic heart disease and the *absence* of concomitant coronary artery disease (CAD) point to a better prognosis. Approximately 48% of all patients undergoing valve surgery have CAD as well. The presence of ischemic heart disease is a serious condition that warrants careful consideration for revascularizing the heart while performing valve replacement/repair to minimize the risk of inhibiting left ventricular (LV) function. Morbidity rates range from 0.1-5.0% depending on the type of complication experienced. In contrast to CABG patients, post valve replacement patients are at an increased risk for thrombosis, thromboembolism or hemorrhage due to prosthetic design or the need to anticoagulate an implanted mechanical (foreign) device. Rates for thrombosis range from 0.1-3.3%. Throm-

TABLE 4. Positive Prognostic Indicators for Patients Undergoing Cardiac Valve Surgery.

Symptoms < 3 years
Functional Class I & II
Age <60
Absence of systemic illness
Etiology of disease
Positive LV function
No previous myocardial infarction

boembolism is most commonly seen in the brain, coronaries, extremities, kidneys, mesentery and retinas, with reported rates of 0.5-3% for aortic valve replacement (AVR) and 0.5-5% for mitral valve replacement (MVR). These rates are influenced by the type of valve utilized as well as the use of proper anticoagulation. Hemorrhage is a well documented potential risk as a result of the need to anticoagulate. Morbidity rates range from 1.3-2.7% with mortality rates of 0.1-0.5%. Central nervous system (CNS) and gastrointestinal (GI) bleeding are associated with the highest instances of mortality. Another unique complication faced by the patient undergoing valve replacement is that of device failure - either as a result of manufacturing defects in mechanical devices or degenerative changes experienced with tissue prostheses. Manufacturing defects, although known to happen, fortunately have a rare rate of occurrence. Incidences of failure usually occur at a rate of 0.003 or less and therefore do not warrant explantation, but rather awareness of the potential for failure and its symptomatology so that both physician and patient can be aware of this risk. Degenerative changes associated with bioprostheses (tissue) continue to plague both the surgeon and the patient, despite the advent of improved manufacturing techniques. Clearly the chance of tissue degeneration increases with time. Reports of 90-95% failure free rates at 6-7 years post implantation are routinely reported, with that same rate decreasing to 70-80% at 10 years. Children, young adults and patients with renal disease - or those that experience an altered calcium metabolism - have increased rates of tissue calcification or fiber degeneration.

TIMING OF SURGERY

As mortality and morbidity rates are well documented, the timing of surgery remains a critical issue. Obviously the goals are to relieve symptoms and increase long term survival, while preventing irreversible LV dysfunction. To improve clinical and functional results, efforts have been directed at improving surgical techniques (i.e., myocardial preservation) or the valve design. However, 20-30% of patients undergoing valve surgery still have suboptimal postoperative outcomes associated with persistent LV enlargement, little or no regression in left ventricular mass and decreased left ventricular systolic function. Therefore determining the timing of cardiac surgical intervention vs. medical treatment becomes a balancing act of weighing the known risks of the procedure vs. the risk of developing irreversible myocardial damage. Table 5 provides a simplistic schema of a decision tree which may be utilized in performing such an act. Patients classified in NYHA classes 3 and 4 may warrant immediate surgical intervention, while those in class 1 and 2 may benefit from further testing and observation that would assess a patient's tolerance for exercise and/or left ventricular function.

TABLE 5. Aortic/Mitral Regurgitation or Stenosis: Determining the Timing of Surgery.

NYHA I-II		NYHA III-IV
↓		↓
EST		Valve Surgery
Good	Poor	
↓	↓	
Assess LV	Valve Surgery	
↓	↓	
Abnormal	Normal	
↓	↓	
Confirm with testing		
↓		
Valve Surgery	Reassess q 6-12 mo.	

TABLE 6. The Ten Commandments of Valve Design.

1. It must not propagate emboli.
2. It must be chemically inert and not damage blood elements.
3. It must offer no resistance to physiological flows.
4. It must close promptly (less than 0.05 second).
5. It must remain closed during the appropriate phase of the cardiac cycle.
6. It must have lasting physical and geometric features.
7. It must be inserted in a physiological site (generally the normal anatomical site).
8. It must be capable of permanent fixation.
9. It must not annoy the patient.
10. It must be technically practical to insert.

From: Harken, DE. Heart Valves: Ten commandments and still counting. *Ann Thorac Surg*, 1989; 48:S18-9. (reprinted with permission)

VALVE DESIGN

In 1950 Dr. Dwight Harken proposed the "Ten Commandments" of valve design (Table 6). His vision was prophetic as these criteria are still applicable today. These commandments can be grouped into 6 criteria that should be considered when looking at valve design and selection; hemodynamics, thrombogenicity, hemolysis, durability, implantability and audibility. Each criteria is critical when considering design and selection of a valve prosthesis. *Hemodynamics* that most closely mimic the function of native valves are most desirable. Valve design is structured to provide smooth/laminar flow with a minimal transvalvular gradient across the orifice. The valve should open easily with negligible resistance and close correctly to prevent regurgitation or backflow of blood. *Thrombogenicity* or the tendency to form blood clot, must be minimized. The use of pyrolytic carbon and similar structural elements has contributed to the reduction of this problem. Devices are configured to minimize any changes in flow or pressure that could contribute to clot formation. *Hemolysis* or the destruction of red blood cells occurs if the blood flow pattern is disturbed. Valve designs are manufactured to minimize this problem as well. *Durability* is obviously of critical importance. Improvements in materials used to manufacture mechanical valves has allowed sustained, consistent performance for this group of devices. As stated previously, tissue valves are still plagued by degradation or tissue breakdown leading to malfunction at an average of 6-10 years post implantation. Valves must be safely, easily and securely implanted. *Implantability* is achieved by the use of a sewing ring that allows a stable tissue-to- prosthesis linkage. Correct sizing is crucial to ensure this link. Finally, the noise the valve makes or its *audibility* should be considered. Although the ability to hear "clicks" are extremely rare in newer valve models, older versions may produce noises disturbing to the patient.

All prostheses can be grouped into two broad categories: mechanical or tissue. Generally, mechanical devices can be classified into one of three types of design: caged-ball (i.e. Starr-Edwards), Tilting-Disc, (Medtronic Hall) or bi-leaflet (St. Jude). These valves are constructed of varying combinations of metal, plastic, dacron, etc. While highly durable and easily implanted, they may be associated with increased rates of hemolysis, and thromboembolism. Anticoagulation must be provided to reduce the risks of these complications. They may also be audible and provide adequate, but not superior hemodynamic performance. Tissue valves are generally constructed of either porcine (i.e. Carpentier-Edwards) or bovine (Ionescu-Shiley) pericardium. Human heart valves harvested from donors are being utilized with increasing frequency as the result of relatively new cryopreservation techniques that allow for prolonged storage with minimal tissue breakdown. While tissue degeneration and calcification remains a significant disadvantage of this category of valve, good hemodynamic performance, low thromboembolism rates and the lack of need to anticoagulate provides distinct advantages for the patient when selecting a type of prosthesis.

Selection of a specific valve for a patient warrants careful consideration of several factors. Patients ability or inability to tolerate the anticoagulation necessary for mechanical valves clearly influences the choice of tissue vs. mechanical valve. In light of this, a patient's compliance (i.e. willingness and ability to consistently take medication), past medical history (i.e. presence of ulcers, history of previous cerebral vascular accident (CVA), and activity level or lifestyle (i.e. involvement in contact sports) should be elicited in order to make an informed choice. The patient's age should be factored in the decision making process as well. As tissue valves are known to degrade or calcify over time, younger patients would appear not to be good choices for this class of valve. Other factors, however might necessitate a need to choose this type of device. In general, tissue valves are a strong option for elderly patients. Finally, cardiac anatomy may also influence valve choice, particularly if the valve must be placed in a small aortic root. Clearly, the decision of the class (tissue vs. mechanical) of valve and specific design is an important one that warrants patient and physician collaboration to select an optimal replacement for the native valve.

POSTOPERATIVE MANAGEMENT

Once the valve has been selected and implanted into the patient via open-heart surgery, unique nursing interventions are performed to manage the valve replacement patient. Nursing assessments and interventions appropriate for the patient undergoing a CABG procedure are also performed with this patient population. As mentioned, several interventions unique to the valve patient should also be carried out. Volume management and assessment of hemodynamics should be carefully considered, particularly in patients with significantly abnormal preoperative pathology that led to valvular dysfunction. Elevated left atrial pressure (LAP), pulmonary artery occlusion pressure (PAOP) and chronic or severe pulmonary artery pressure (PAP) are not uncommon and reflect the heart's attempt to compensate for the changes in blood flow that occurred because of the disease process. Subsequently, volume resuscitation should be administered with extra caution. Stenotic lesions and hypertrophied cavities may require *less* volume, while regurgitant processes and dilated cavities may require *more* volume. *Arrhythmias* are more commonly seen in the valve patient than in the patient undergoing CABG, as the electrical pathways of the heart are anatomically located near the valve structures. Inadvertent surgical injury or edema (swelling) of tissue secondary to manipulation may result in heart blocks or irritability. For these reasons, pacing wires are routinely placed in this patient population as an added tool to manage the problem should it develop. Heart sounds are critical in the post valve replacement patient. Obtaining an accurate baseline immediately after surgery, may assist the health care team in assessing cardiac function. Specifically, a new onset murmur previously not detected warrants physician notification and additional follow up. Also, the presence of absence of a "click" should be noted. As previously stated, all valves do not produce an audible click. Absence of a click on admission with subsequent development of one in the later phase of recovery does not generally represent a problem. Rather, the sound simply might have been masked by the noises generated from mechanical ventilation, mediastinal tubes and fluid in the mediastinal space. However, presence of a click on admission that can no longer be heard indeed may be a sign of thrombus formation and should be brought to a physician's attention. Neurological assessment is performed as one would for any open heart patient with an added emphasis on a return to pre-operative baseline CNS function. Because of the increased risk for dislodgement of emboli formed from calcified and/or vegetative valves, post valve replacement patients experience a higher risk for sustaining a cerebral event in contrast to the CABG patient.

The following questions may be used as a guide to elicit information specific to a valve patient, that in turn, will allow the nurse to anticipate patients' needs.

1. What process caused the need for surgery?
2. Which valve(s) was affected?
3. Was the process chronic or acute?
4. What surgical procedure was used?
5. Which prosthesis was selected?

CARDIAC VALVE REPAIR

Cardiac valve repair has recently experienced a resurgence of interest as the "ideal" prosthesis has yet to be developed. The efficacy of repair vs. replacement is still controversial, however lingering problems with tissue valve durability and thromboembolism rates associated with mechanical valves has led to a trend of increased numbers of valve repairs being performed. Commissurotomy procedures to open stenosed valves, or annuloplasty to tighten "floppy" valves are still classic operative techniques used to repair specific defects. However, more extensive repair work is now being performed in an effort to save the native valve. Currently, repair work is primarily limited to the mitral valve. The anatomic design of this valve best lends itself to repair work. Because of this, patient selection is typically focused on those experiencing mitral insufficiency secondary to ruptured chordae. Certain anatomic considerations must be reviewed when attempting repair. The mitral valve is composed of 2 leaflets; anterior (aortic) and posterior. The aortic leaflet possesses the shortest of arc of annular attachment (3-5 cm) but occupies two thirds of the orifice area, with the posterior leaflet attaching to the remainder of the annulus. Any reconstruction that does not involve decreasing the area of the anterior leaflet will generally achieve a positive result as long as its mobility is protected. Particular care must be exercised when performing repair work on this valve as critical structures (i.e. left circumflex coronary artery, bundle of His) run close to the valve.

A variety of surgical repair procedures are currently being performed. Patching of localized perforations, and a variety of methods to stabilize, and tighten valve structures are possible with better results being reported for work on the posterior leaflet. Although results vary from institution to institution, this appears to be a promising avenue for treating specific valvular dysfunction. Clearly more data is necessary before conclusions can be drawn.

SUMMARY

Cardiac valvular surgery continues to present unique and exciting challenges for the health care team. Prevention of disease, precise timing of surgery, improved prosthesis design and surgical innovations are leading to favorable outcomes for this patient population.

INTRAOPERATIVE CARE OF THE CABG PATIENT:

A NURSING DIAGNOSIS APPROACH

Gail Kaempf, R.N., MSN, CNOR

Presbyterian Medical Center of Philadelphia
Philadelphia, Pennsylvania

This section addresses intraoperative nursing interventions for adult patients undergoing uncomplicated coronary artery bypass grafting (CABG). Nursing diagnoses for this patient population will be identified and discussed. The objectives for the participant are to describe basic components of the CABG procedure and to identify nursing diagnoses and intraoperative interventions for the adult patient undergoing CABG.

A nursing diagnosis is an actual or potential health problem. It focuses on the human response of an individual or a group. The nurse identifies the problem and then treats it independently. Collaborative problems focus on pathophysiologic response. Nurses identify these problems and work inter-dependently with other team members. Both nursing diagnoses and collaborative problems are incorporated into the care of the patient.

Coronary artery bypass grafting (CABG) is a surgical technique for improving myocardial blood flow in patients with ischemic heart disease. This involves a median sternotomy and the use of cardiopulmonary bypass.(CPB) The area of the coronary artery obstruction is bypassed with a graft. The coronary arteries distal to the area of obstruction need to be normal. A CABG procedure is usually performed where there is obstruction of a vessel greater than 50-70%.

Physical improvement for the patient due to surgical intervention has been shown to be beneficial. Califf et al[1] published their results in 1989, looking at 5809 patients that were treated for coronary artery disease over 15 years. There were 2847 treated medically, 2663 were treated with the CABG within 6 months of the cardiac catheterization, and 299 were treated with the CABG after 6 months of medical treatment. Patients with more extensive coronary artery disease and those

Cardiac Surgery: Current Issues, Edited by A.C. Cernaianu
and A.J. DelRossi Plenum Press, New York, 1992

with greater decrease in ventricular function had the greatest improvement in five year post surgery. In 1984, the five year survival rate with CABG was significantly better than five year survival rate with medical therapy.

Myers et al[2] published their results in 1989 from a six year follow-up of 1,921 patients treated surgically and 679 patients treated medically for coronary artery disease. Patients had 70% stenosis of three coronary arteries. The results showed that patients with proximal lesions had a 40% survival rate when treated medically and an 81% survival rate when treated surgically. Patients with severe left ventricular dysfunction who were treated medically had a 30% survival rate compared with 63% for those treated surgically. Early operation was a strong predictor of survival.

Hochberg et al[3] compared the clinical outcome of 125 percutaneus transluminal coronary angioplasty (PTCA) patients to 125 CABG patients. These were patients who had single or double vessel disease. Eighty-eight percent of the PTCA patients were successful initially with 14 late deaths. One-hundred twenty-four out of 125 CABG procedures were successful with two late deaths. After three years, 63% of the patients having PTCA and 92% of the patients having CABG procedures were alive. Nineteen percent of the original PTCAs required CABG during the three year study period.

A frequently identified nursing diagnosis for patients undergoing CABG is anxiety related to the fear of the unknown and death. It is important to take time to speak with the patient and the patient's family members and significant others about their concerns and their understanding of the surgery and it's implications as well as what are the patient's methods of coping with the situation. The nurse needs to review the past medical history, including previous surgery, the existence of chronic illness, allergies, and patient's current medications, and the laboratory values. The perioperative nurse should begin the intraoperative plan with the patient and the family members to help relieve their anxiety and while also building rapport with them. Patient and family education is an important aspect at this time.

Raleigh, Lepczyk, and Rowley[4] studied the benefit of preoperative information for significant others. The authors found that significant others were more anxious than patients prior to receiving all necessary information. Although after the class, the significant other's average anxiety decreased, it still remained at higher level close to that of the patient. Significant other's anxiety may be induced by a high degree of helplessness. The spouses and relatives face a potential crisis when a family member is undergoing CABG surgery and they also need to be incorporated into the plan of care. Families have identified that waiting during surgery and the recovery room time as the worst time of the hospitalization. Norheim,[5] studied 68 subjects undergoing elective, first-time CABG surgeries. The questionaire included an inventory list of 45 needs. Subjects were asked to participate while they were in the waiting room 3½-4 hours after the patient left for surgery. The highest ranking need noted was to have questions answered honestly. The second highest need was to be reassured that the best care was being given to the patient. The third highest ranking need was to feel there was hope. Thirty-nine percent of the subjects indicated that nurses provided the most help during the operative period, followed by physicians at 27%, other relatives 8%, religious advisors 8%, and friends at 7%. Of the top 21 needs identified and shared by spouses and relatives, 14 were concerned with the need for obtaining information. Families wanted to know whether complications developed during surgery. They needed time to mobilize their crisis-meeting resources. More frequent reports on the patient's progress during the surgery might help families better cope with the stress of waiting. Nurses need to provide the opportunities for spouses to talk about the possibility of the patient's death. Subjects indicated that the need for more information about the patient's progress in surgery is a very important need that is not being met. A clinical nurse specialist is a valuable adjunct in strengthening the crisis-meeting resources of spouses and relatives. This allows for one nurse to coordinate pre - and postoperative teaching to ensure continuity of care.

Once the perioperative nurse has completed her preoperative assessment she is ready to plan her care for the operative phase. Much activity occurs in the operating room prior to the entry of the patient. Personnel from the anesthesia team check their equipment. They access lines on the patient, and once the patient is in the room they monitor the patient with an electrocardiogram machine. During this time, also, the perfusionist primes the heart-lung machine. There is much activity on the part of the perioperative nurses to prepare for the procedure and patient care. Observation is the key. Anticipation in preparing for the needs of the patient, surgical team, and anesthesia team is paramount. There are many nursing diagnoses at this time which are similar to those utilized in other areas of nursing. Potential for infection is a concern. The body's protective barrier is violated intraoperatively and it is essential to practice aseptic technique. Potential impairment of skin integrity is another consideration. Kemp et al,[6] published their results in 1990. They looked at 125 patients undergoing a variety of surgical procedures. Fifteen patients developed a total of 23 pressure sores. Sixteen pressure sores were rated as Stage I, 6 pressure sores as Stage II, and one pressure sore as Stage III. By day 10 of discharge, 14 of the 23 pressure sores (61%) had resolved. The most common site included elbows, heels and sacrum. It was found that extracorporeal circulation coupled with age and time on the operating room table were predictors for the development of 12 of the 15 patients with pressure sores; 83 of 110 patients remained pressure sore free.

Potential for injury, due to the patient's altered level of consciousness and unfamiliarity with the operating room environment is a constant consideration. As the circulating nurse introduces her/himself, patient identification and procedure are verified. Patient anxiety is elevated as the patient is wheeled into the operating room and sees machinery and instrumentation. Another anxiety stimulus is the number of personnel in the operating room preparing and caring for the patient. It is important to note that the time span for the patient leaving her/his room until the actual incision in the operating room may be up to 90 minutes. Family members often envision the start for incision occurring soon after the patient was taken from her/his room. Informing the family of the start time may allay some of the anxiety. At this time also, patient comfort is essential since increasing the patient's stress may increase the heart's need for oxygen. Warm blankets are usually appreciated by the patient. Checking to make sure that emergency equipment such as the defibrillator, external pacemaker, and extra blood in the operating room refrigerator are available is important preparation. In order to keep anesthesia and cardiopulmonary bypass time to a minimum, all equipment needed during the procedure should be readily accessible.

Once anesthetized and intubated, the patient is positioned for surgical access. Maintenance of hemodynamic status and protection of bony prominences/compromised skin areas is promoted. Foley or rectal temperature probe, Foley catheter, and electrosurgical unit pad are placed. The patient is prepped and draped. Sternotomy and retrieval of the saphenous vein are performed simultaneously. Potential for infection related to wound contamination from the leg incision to the sternum is a concern. Instruments used on the leg are kept separate from those used in the chest. The length of the saphenous vein to be harvested is determined by the number of grafts that will be needed, i.e. approximately 20 cm per graft. An incision is made on the medial aspect of the leg, the vein is mobilized, the branches are tied and clipped, and the vein is removed. The vein is checked to insure patency and repairs are made to prevent leakage. Once the chest incision is made, an electrocautery is used to cut through the tissue and to provide hemostasis. A saw is used for sternotomy. If the internal mammary artery is used, then a special retractor is secured to the side of the table. The left side of the chest is elevated as the internal mammary artery lies right under the sternum. Papaverine may be used to prevent arterial spasm and dilate the artery. Dissection of the internal mammary artery takes longer, is also somewhat more difficult, and patients tend to have more chest pain postoperatively. Wound infection is more common in patients with bilateral IMA grafts, and this is attributable to diabetes or advanced age.

In patients where the internal mammary artery (IMA) grafts are used, a 90 percent patency rate has been obtained 7-10 years postoperative, as opposed to the saphenous vein grafts which have been related to a rate of 40-50 percent closure within 10 years. Of the 50-70 percent remaining grafts that are open, there has been greater than 50 percent stenosis. Once the IMA is available, the retractors removed and the sternal retractor applied, pericardial stitches are anchored and the heart is exposed for the surgical procedure. The patient is heparinized systemically, Cannulation stitches are placed followed by the cannulae. It is important that there is no air in the arterial system. Patients are put on bypass after the vein is ready. Circulatory bypass or extracorporeal circulation is a method of maintaining near normal hemodynamic and metabolic conditions in living organisms during a temporary absence of cardiac and pulmonary function. It involves three components, the pump, oxygenator, and plastic circuitry. Blood is routed from the right atrium to the heart lung machine and back to the body via aortic cannula. The circulatory bypass oxygenates and cools blood, thereby lowering body temperature. Cooling of the temperature down to 28°C to 32°C decreases normal tissue oxygen requirements. When the patient is cold enough, the heart will stop and may still fibrillate. Therefore, a cardioplegic solution is infused into the aortic root at temperatures anywhere from 4°C to 20°C. A main ingredient in the cardioplegic solution is potassium. This will stop the fibrillation. Also, cold saline may be applied topically to aid in cooling the heart. It is important to correlate the temperatures of solutions that are used in the body with the temperature of the blood and solution circulated by the pump.

Currently, 3-7 percent of patients who have CABG procedures need re-operation. Sternotomy may produce massive hemorrhage, thus, it is important that extra blood is readily available. Prolonged bleeding can be a problem, especially after discontinuation of bypass. Usually fresh frozen plasma and platelets are ordered prior to surgery and administered after the patient is off bypass. Perioperative MI may be encountered because of potential embolization of old vein graft atheroma. A more recent study shows that there may be no significant differences in overall operative morbidity rates or specific surgical complications for the initial repeat CABGs. Long-term results of redo CABG are not quite as good as the primary procedure, although they are close.[7]

Once the patient is on bypass and cooled down to an appropriate level, the distal grafts are begun. Distal grafts involve those that are sewn directly onto the heart muscle, proximal grafts are those that are sewn onto the aorta. In situations where the IMA is used, the proximal graft does not need to be done because the IMA is still connected to it's origin. The vein is reversed prior to sewing onto the heart to prevent the valves from obstructing the flow of blood. Again the vein is checked for leaks and is repaired prior to use. After the site for anastomosis is selected, the dissection of the coronary artery follows. The anastomosis is performed with fine suture, usually 6-0 or 7-0 Prolene. The anastomosis is completed; cardioplegic solution is circulated through the site to insure that the anastomosis is complete. When the last distal graft is started rewarming of the patient is begun. Proximal grafts are sewn onto the aorta. The cross clamp is removed and a partial occlusion clamp is applied in order for the aortotomy to be performed. Warm saline is used during this period. As the body temperature increases, the nurse should closely watch the monitor for ventricular fibrillation. One must be prepared to use the defibrillator. After the proximal grafts are completed, the partial occlusion clamp is removed. When the patient's venous temperature is 37°C-38°C, the patient is weaned off of bypass. During this time, temporary pacing wires are sewn onto the heart and the chest tubes are placed in the mediastinal area. If the pleural cavity has been entered, as in the case when the internal mammary artery graft is utilized, extra chest tubes are placed and connected to the chest tube drainage system. The surgical area is checked for hemostasis. Antibiotic solution is used to irrigate the chest after removal of the cannulae. The chest is closed in anatomic layers. Dressings are applied to the chest and leg incisions.

The instrument tables are kept sterile until after the patient leaves the room, in the event that the patient should undergo an emergency re-entry. The circulating nurse communicates to the nurse in the Intensive Care Unit as to the patient's history, allergies, current medication, status during the operative procedure, what the operative procedure was and any specific requirements that the patient may have. Documentation is an important component of patient care. By understanding the surgical procedure, the perioperative nurse can better anticipate needs in order to expedite the procedure, be prepared for potential problems, and provide better quality patient care.

One of the advances in cardiac surgery is the use of the right gastroepiploic artery (RGEA) for use in patients needing coronary artery bypass surgery. This is useful in patients in whom vein grafts are of poor quality or when the veins have been removed earlier, and in patients with severely calcified ascending aortas where no anastomosis of the proximal graft onto the aorta is possible. One advantage of the RGEA is that it does not interfere with sternal blood supply, as happens with the use of the internal mammary artery. There are contraindications for this particular procedure. Patients with previous laparotomies present difficulty in dissection. There is higher frequency of postoperative bleeding associated with this procedure. Also, severe obesity and history of abdominal illness with probable necessity for future laparotomy also represent contraindications. When a second laparotomy is indicated, it is important for the surgeon to have knowledge of the previous RGEA anastomoses to prevent operative injury. There are technical considerations with this procedure. The artery is marked when it is harvested to prevent twisting. Papaverine and saline are introduced to prevent spasm. Various routes to the diaphragm are available. The pedicle graft is generally thicker than the IMA graft, however this has no adverse effect. Long-term results are not yet available. Mills and Everson[8] published their results in 1989. They followed 39 patients where 41 RGEA grafts and 43 concomitant IMA grafts were used. Fifteen were free grafts and 26 pedicles. Six of the patients had no vein grafts. Early postoperative cardiac catheterizations showed that all RGEA grafts were patent without kinks. Three free grafts had vasospasm. Verkkala[9] and his group published their results in 1989. They anastomosed the RGEA to the right coronary artery and the IMA to the LAD and circumflex artery. Postoperative coronary angiography showed a patent RGEA in 82 percent of the subjects. One patient had occlusion of the graft and hepatomegaly.

It is evident from recent data that the physical condition of the patient undergoing surgical myocardial revascularization has been greatly improved. Allen,[10] in 1990, reviewed the literature, looking at the physical and psychosocial outcomes after CABG. The majority of patients (70-90%) experienced relief from angina. Exercise performance increased 20 to 50 percent after surgery. It is interesting to note that, although the physical findings were quite dramatic, the psychosocial effects may have lasting effects and may represent a challenge to the nurse. Fifty percent of the patients experienced psychiatric symptoms. Most of them presented with depression, however, with no psychiatric symptoms while in the hospital. Most of these patients became less self-reliant, more socially constricted and had decreased expression of sexual and aggressive drives after surgery. One-third encountered significant psychologic obstacles to recovery, lasting up to one year post surgery. This included anxiety and somatic preoccupation. Approximately 80 percent of the patients reported a decrease in employment. Preoperative work status may be a major predictor for postoperative employment. A period of inactivity greater than 6 months before CABG surgery resulted in a 50 percent chance of inactivity postoperatively. In general, male patients younger than 55 years and those with a higher income preoperatively, are more likely to return to work. This poses a challenge to all nurses. Outcomes of CABG surgery are more effective than medical treatment in relieving angina, increasing exercise tolerance, and decreasing short-term need for anti-anginal medications. Full resumption of social and leisure activities and return to work for most CABG patients has not been demonstrated. Preoperative levels of functional status can deteriorate after surgery. Information from the studies presented and future studies should enable the nurse to systematically do predischarge planning and counseling. Although great achievements have been made in enhancing physiologic outcomes, nursing needs to address psychological issues to better enable patients to return to a more functional level in their community.

REFERENCES

1. R.M. Califf, F.E. Harrell,Jr., K.L. Lee, J.S. Rankin, M.A. Haltky, D.B. Mark, R.H. Jones, L.H. Muhlbaier, H.N. Oldham, Jr., D.B. Pryor: The evolution of medical and surgical therapy for coronary artery disease:a 15-year perspective. *JAMA*, 261:2077-86;1989.

2. W.O. Myers, H.V. Schaff, B.J. Gersh, L.D. Fisher, A.S. Kosinski, M.B. Mock, D.R. Holmes, T.J. Ryan, G.Z. Kaiser and Cass Investigators: Improved survival of surgically treated patients with triple vessel coronary artery disease and severe angina pectoris: A report from the coronary artery study (CASS) registry. *J Thorac Cardiovasc Surg* 97:487-95;1989.
3. M.S. Hochberg, I. Gielchinsky, V. Parsonnet, S.M. Hussain, E. Mirosky, D. Fisch: Coronary angioplasty versus coronary bypass: Three year follow-up of a matched series of 250 patients. *J Thorac Cardiovasc* Surg 97:496-503;1989.
4. E.H. Raleigh, M. Lepczyk, C. Rowley: Significant others benefit from preoperative information. *J Adv Nurs* 15(8):941-45;1990.
5. C. Norheim: Family needs of patients having coronary artery bypass graft surgery during the intraoperative period. *Heart & Lung*, 18(6):622-26;1989.
6. M.G. Kemp, J.K. Keithley, D.W. Smith, B. Morreale: Factors that contribute to pressure sores in surgical patients. *Res Nurs Health* 13:293-301;1990.
7. M.H. Franey, K. Gabel, D.E. Berg: Re-operation: Cardiac surgery. AACN Clinical Issues: *Crit Care Nurs* 1(1):72-78;1990.
8. N.L. Mills, C.T. Everson: Right gastroepiploic artery: A third arterial conduit for coronary artery bypass. *Ann Thorac Surg*, 47:706-11;1989.
9. K. Verkkala, A. Jarvinen, P. Keto, K. Virtanen, A. Lehtola, T. Pellinen: Right gastroepiploic artery as a coronary bypass graft. *Ann of Thorac Surg* 47:716-719;1989.
10. J.K. Allen: Physical and psychosocial outcomes after coronary artery bypass graft surgery: Review of the Literature. *Heart & Lung* 19(1):49-54;1990.

ECMO: AN OVERVIEW FOR PERFUSIONISTS

Mark Kurusz, C.C.P.

Department of Surgery
Division of Cardiothoracic Surgery
The University of Texas Medical Branch
Galveston, Texas

While virtually all perfusionists have heard about extracorporeal membrane oxygenation (ECMO) and perhaps been tested on it as part of their certification exam, few have been directly involved with it until recently. It also only peripherally relates to cardiac surgery, but use of ECMO after open-heart surgery or as a bridge-to-transplantation represents a small but growing field. While ECMO is conceptually similar to the more familiar cardiopulmonary bypass practiced in the operating room, there are some fundamental differences.

Both obviously rely on an artificial lung and mechanical pump to support the patient's cardiopulmonary requirements, and many of the technical aspects are familiar to perfusionists. But one of the most incredible aspects of ECMO is that patients, primarily newborns, can be connected to an extracorporeal circuit, systemically anticoagulated

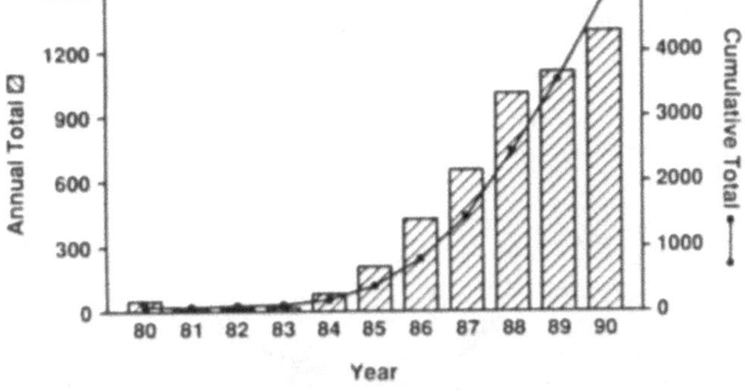

Figure 1. Neonatal annual and cumulative totals, 1973-1990. (Courtesy Extracorporeal Life Support Organization, Ann Arbor, Michigan, October 1991)

and supported for not one or two hours, but days or even weeks, and still survive. There are a growing number of "success stories" regarding ECMO, and patients treated to date now number in the several thousand.

Figure 1 illustrates the dramatic growth in the number of neonatal ECMO patients from programs in the United States and abroad who voluntarily send in registry reports on their patients to the Extracorporeal Life Support Organization (ELSO) at Ann Arbor, Michigan. The first bar represents eight years between 1973 and 1980 when a total of 48 patients were done. Until 1984, the number of neonates treated with ECMO still was modest; by the end of 1990, however, nearly 5000 patients have been treated, and the growth, while doubling each year in the mid 1980s, has averaged about 15% per year for the last three years. Therefore, ECMO is clearly an area of tremendous growth, in contrast to open-heart surgery which has tended to plateau in recent years due to the fact that other procedures such as percutaneous transluminal coronary angioplasty have evolved for treatment of coronary artery disease.

Perfusionists should be involved in ECMO for many reasons, not the least of which are the statistics shown in Figure 1. While some have expressed concerns to the fact that perfusion has "lost" ECMO to other allied health specialties, this chapter will describe how perfusionists can participate in the success of this remarkable technology.[1]

This chapter will briefly review some of the historical mileposts in the clinical applications of ECMO, outline the medical indications, and summarize the most recent collective results from the ELSO database. Logistical and technical aspects, including complications of the procedure will be described based on the author's experience at an ECMO center since 1987. Finally, a review of future directions of ECMO which have been speculated about by those in the field will be outlined.

WHAT IS ECMO?

ECMO denotes temporary, prolonged extracorporeal membrane oxygenation for acute, severe, reversible respiratory and/or cardiac failure. Excellent review articles have been published [2-4] as well as a

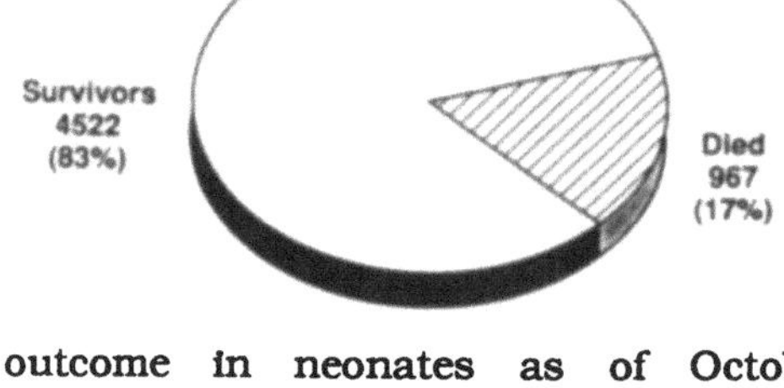

Figure 2. ECMO outcome in neonates as of October, 1991. (Courtesy Extracorporeal Life Support Organization, Ann Arbor, Michigan, October 1991)

technical manual[5] describing the most commonly used methodology for ECMO.

Historically, extracorporeal oxygenation for respiratory failure in a newborn was first attempted in Philadelphia by Rashkind and co-workers[6] in the 1960s. It was not called ECMO then, probably because they used a bubble oxygenator. This team's approach relied on the patient's femoral arterial blood pressure to drive blood through a primitive, custom-made device, and the mode was arterio-venous. Ten patients were treated: four were children with cystic fibrosis, who were artificially oxygenated for up to 8 hours; four were newborns with respiratory distress syndrome and were supported for 1, 12, 16, and 27 hours, respectively; two others were supported during open-heart surgery. Only one of the cardiac surgery patients survived after extra-corporeal oxygenation for one hour with this so-called "pumpless" technique. All patients, however, improved with the device and the rate of hemolysis was extremely low. It is important to stress that the underlying irreversible pulmonary disease was the cause of death in the non-survivors.

In 1972, Hill and co-workers[7] reported the first successful prolonged extracorporeal membrane oxygenation case which was in an adult. A 24-year-old man was involved in an automobile accident and had multiple trauma. Four days later he developed the so-called "shock-lung syndrome," despite the appropriation of conventional management. He was placed on femoral vein to femoral artery extracorporeal support using bi-directional cannulae in both vessels. A Bramson membrane oxygenator was used, and he was supported for 75 hours at a bypass flow of between 3 and 3.6 L/minute. Ventilator settings were decreased, the shock-lung syndrome reversed, and the patient recovered. A second successful case for pulmonary fat embolism was included in Hill's original report as an addendum. In both cases, the extracorporeal circuit provided approximately 50 to 75% of the systemic blood flow. The hematocrit was maintained between 30 and 37%, but the platelet count was markedly decreased and had to be corrected with frequent infusions of platelets.

This was followed by clinical trials in infants by Bartlett and co-workers[8] at the University of California, Irvine. The first successful case in this series was a 36-hour long cardiac support in a 2 year-old after a Mustard procedure. The first neonate to survive was a 3.4 kg full-term female with persistent fetal circulation. She was put on ECMO 18 hours after birth and supported for seven days, during which time a patent ductus arteriosus was ligated. This case and others performed by Dr. Bartlett's group demonstrated the feasibility of the technique in neonates.

A multicenter prospective randomized trial of ECMO in 90 adults with acute respiratory failure was reported in 1979.[9] The survival rate with ECMO was 9.5% compared with 8.3% using conventional ventilatory management. This led to a general disinterest in the technique for adults.

Table 1. Neonatal ECMO outcome by primary respiratory diagnosis.

DIAGNOSIS	TOTAL	SURVIVAL %
MAS	2067	93
CDH	996	61
RDS/HMD	788	85
SEPSIS	752	77
PPHN/PFC	692	88
ALS	22	59

MAS=meconium aspiration syndrome; CDH=congenital diaphragmatic hernia; RDS=respiratory distress syndrome; HMD=hyaline membrane disease; PPHN=persistent pulmonary hypertension in the newborn; PFC=persistent fetal circulation; ALS=air leak syndrome. (Courtesy Extracorporeal Life Support Organization, Ann Arbor, Michigan, October 1991)

Tremendous improvements have been made in the last decade. Figure 2 depicts the current international survival statistics for neonates treated with ECMO as of October, 1991. There are now 5,479 cases reported in the ELSO Registry from 79 centers. Eighty-three percent of the patients have survived, and ECMO is now considered standard therapy for term newborns with severe respiratory failure unresponsive to maximum medical management.[10] There are currently 70 ECMO programs in the United States and 12 in other countries listed as institutional members of ELSO. Figure 3 illustrates the growth in the number of centers by year beginning in 1982. Note the tremendous increase in 1987 when the number of centers doubled to 45 total.

WHY PERFORM ECMO?

ECMO should not be applied unless the respiratory and/or cardiac

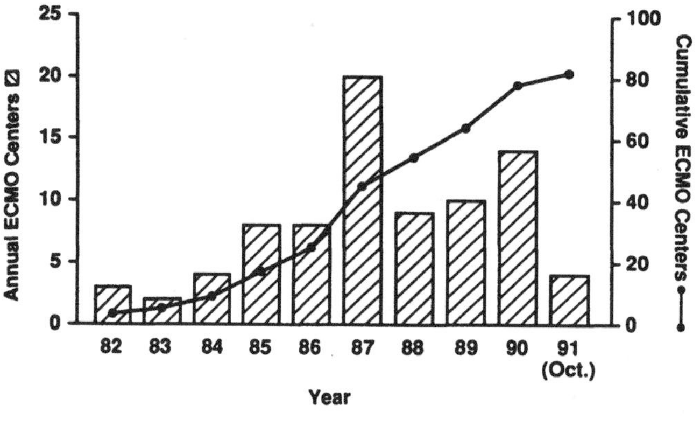

Figure 3. ECMO centers by year, 1982-1991. (Courtesy Extracorporeal Life Support Organization, Ann Arbor, Michigan, October 1991)

failure is believed to be reversible during the anticipated period of ECMO support. That is the standard definition, and the neonatal population has been the group treated in greatest numbers. However, there is a small, but growing, patient population treated with ECMO which includes those classified as in need for cardiac support, pediatric respiratory failure, or adult combined respiratory and cardiac dysfunction. Patients who have been on a mechanical ventilator longer than 14 days generally are excluded because of barotrauma.

Contraindications for ECMO in the neonatal age group are as follows: birthweight less than 2 kg or 34 weeks' gestation because of the increased risk of intracranial hemorrhage with systemic anticoagulation. Severe irreversible brain or other organ damage are contraindications. Any bleeding problem that would likely be uncontrollable or life-threatening with heparin anticoagulation is also a contraindication. An intracranial ultrasound is done on all neonates before ECMO to rule out intraventricular hemorrhage that, like the previous criterion, would be aggravated by systemic heparinization. Similarly, any severe underlying non-pulmonary disease must be ruled out. A cardiac echocardiography is also performed as part of the screening because some babies may have a congenital cardiac anomaly which would not be cured by ECMO. Finally, if the pulmonary disease is not expected to resolve within ten days, the patient should not undergo ECMO.

Table 1 depicts the primary respiratory diagnoses and the number of neonatal patients treated as of October, 1991. The most common indication is meconium aspiration syndrome (MAS). More than one-third of the patients are in this category and 93% survived. Congenital diaphragmatic hernia (CDH) is a more difficult problem because most of these babies, in addition to lung hypoplasia and persistent fetal circulation, have had the added stress of a surgical procedure for repair of the hernia. The overall survival rate was 61%. In the respiratory distress syndrome (RDS) (a broad term that includes babies with hyaline membrane disease), an 85% survival rate has been obtained. In patients with sepsis, or those with pneumonia, the survival rate is 77%. Persistent fetal circulation (PFC), sometimes called primary pulmonary hypertension in the newborn (PPHN), had an 88% survival rate. The last category includes a small number of babies with air leak syndrome (ALS), and the survival, like those treated with congenital diaphragmatic hernia, is about 60%.

The mean age of neonates put on ECMO is 49 hours ± 48 hrs, (SD). The average total hours on ECMO is 134 ± 80 hrs, (SD). While non-survivors are typically on slightly longer than those who survive, time of support has never been a reliable predictor of survival.

Several criteria are used by centers to decide when to put a patient on ECMO. The most common is simply, "failure to respond to conventional medical management" with optimum ventilator manipulations which have led to no improvement in the patient's condition. Our program, and about 25% of the others, use the Oxygenation Index (OI) which is derived by multiplying the mean airway pressure by the percent oxygen divided by a post ductal PaO_2. In normal patients this value is zero. If the OI is 20, there is a 50% predicted mortality. If the OI is greater than 40 on two or three consecutive blood gases, the predicted mortality is 80%, and ECMO is warranted. Virtually, all criteria used by other programs predict similarly poor prognoses.

There are other categories of ECMO patient populations listed in the ELSO Registry which are summarized as follows: 489 patients have been put on ECMO for cardiac support, 88% after open-heart surgery and most often following repair of congenital defects. Forty-six percent of these patients have survived. The average age at the time of ECMO in this group was 13 months, with a mean duration of support of 125 hours ± 84 hours, (SD).

A total of 285 pediatric patients have been placed on ECMO for respiratory support with an overall 47% survival rate. The most common diagnosis in this group is viral pneumonia, and the mean age is 33 months ± 49 months. Unlike the neonatal or cardiac group, the duration of ECMO in the pediatric respiratory group is about 10 days, or 245 hours ± 165 hours, (SD). This statistic presents added demands on the ECMO circuit and will be discussed shortly.

The ECMO experience with adults has been limited; they account for less than 1% of all patients in the ELSO Registry to date. It is likely that more than 44 adult patients nationwide have been put on ECMO, but the ELSO database only reflects the number of adults reported by established ECMO centers who participate in ELSO. Three-quarters of these patients needed ECMO for respiratory failure, most often for adult respiratory distress syndrome (ARDS). The other 25% were put on ECMO for cardiac support, most often either before or after cardiac transplantation. The survival statistics for adult ECMO is 43%, their average age is 34 years, and the average duration of support is approximately 200 hours.

Having reviewed the indications for ECMO and the results, it would be appropriate to consider some of the differences between ECMO and conventional cardiopulmonary bypass. The first distinction is that ECMO is highly labor intensive. During a recent 12-month period at our hospital, there were 304 cardiopulmonary bypass cases; the average pump time was 140 minutes, and the total "on pump" time for the year was about 40,000 minutes, or 711 hours. In contrast, 27 ECMO patients were done during the same time frame. The average duration of ECMO support was 205 hours with a total "on pump" time of 5500 hours. These 27 ECMO patients required nearly eight times the number of hours of pump management than did more than 300 open-heart cases. Therefore, a primary logistical consideration is that the perfusion team *cannot cover* the ECMO shifts in addition to their operating room duties.

Now, what level of involvement should there be with the perfusionists if an ECMO program is to be started in a hospital? We have

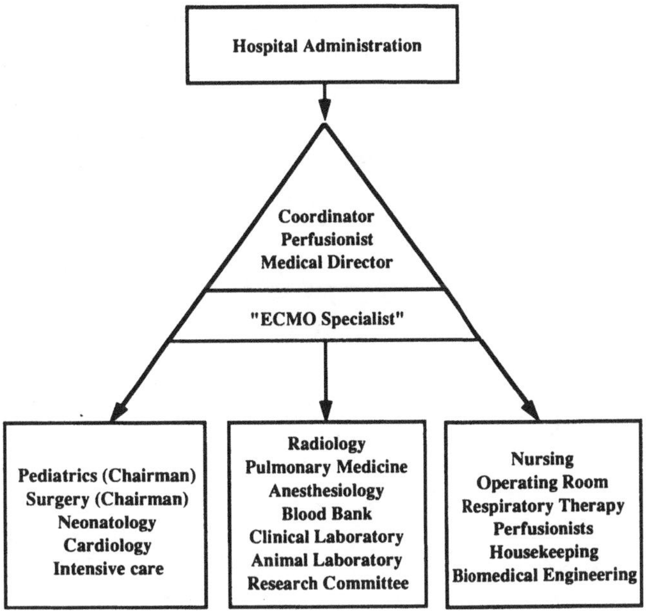

Figure 4. Organization of an ECMO team.

evolved to the organizational structure shown in Figure 4. The central administrative group is composed of three disciplines: the ECMO Nurse Coordinator, the Chief Perfusionist, and the ECMO Medical Director. We have dubbed this the "ECMO triumvirate." These three people have met regularly since the inception of our program to discuss ECMO issues and ensure that adequate communication is maintained. The team has also been responsible for training critical care nurses to become "ECMO Specialists," shown at the bottom of the triangle. ECMO Specialists manage the circuit whenever a patient undergoes ECMO and such management is governed by formal protocols and daily orders determined by the responsible physician.

There is a variety of organizational options used by other programs. However, there is general agreement that physicians, nurses, perfusionists, and respiratory therapists must work together to ensure a successful ECMO team. Nearly all hospital departments and services are affected by the decision to establish an ECMO program. It is very important that good organization and preplanning occur if an ECMO program is to be established in a hospital. In our center we have adopted the policy where the perfusionists are responsible for setting up and priming the ECMO circuit. They are also responsible for providing expertise should an oxygenator need to be changed, or for any other technical problems that may arise. The perfusionists have also provided advice regarding circuit design, including the best equipment and types of monitoring to use, and the development of protocols and checklists in conjunction with the ECMO Coordinator.

What is the role of the ECMO Coordinator and ECMO Nurse Specialist? We patterned our program, as have most others, after the model established at the University of Michigan. Critical care nurses predominate both as coordinators and specialists in all programs in the United States. The coordinator must interact and establish good working relationships with the hospital departments and services, and the coordinator is the one most responsible for the smooth acceptance of ECMO.

Toomasian and Bartlett[11] have emphasized the need for one person with final authority whenever ECMO is performed. Rule by committee in the management of an ECMO patient has many drawbacks. Difficult decisions are sometimes required in any ECMO program regarding termination of treatment, or even the decision as to when to put a baby on. The daily medical problems these patients present are best handled by a physician who acts as medical director.

Odell and colleagues[12] recently surveyed 63 active ECMO centers in the United States to determine team composition and what professions were represented and functioning as ECMO Specialists. About half of the centers reported that their teams were composed of Registered Nurses (RN) exclusively. The second major group had RNs and Registered Respiratory Therapists. Seventeen percent reported combination teams which included physicians assistants, emergency medical technicians, and perfusion assistants functioning as the ECMO Specialist. Four programs had respiratory therapists exclusively, and one program had perfusionists exclusively.

When asked for specific numbers according to specialty, the following results were reported: nurses comprised the largest group and accounted for nearly three-quarters of the total; next were respiratory therapists at 22%. There were 29 perfusionists which accounted for 2%, and there were 44 "other" personnel as mentioned previously. Most interesting, the total number designated as ECMO Specialists in this national survey was 1,431. One can philosophize, debate, and speculate on why perfusionists are not more involved than these figures clearly show. However, these figures are highly accurate and corroborate earlier survey data published in 1990.[13]

The only caution in concluding that perfusionists are minimally involved with ECMO is a previous unpublished survey by Dennis Rivard at Johns Hopkins University. He found that, while few perfusionists functioned as the ECMO Specialist, in about half of the programs, there was perfusion team involvement to the extent that the perfusionists set up and primed the ECMO circuit and were available on a consultative basis. (D. Rivard, personal communication.)

For most cases the duration of ECMO is technically uncomplicated and routine. Servo-regulation and monitoring devices on the ECMO circuit, as well as the fact that the patients are maintained normothermic with no cardiotomy suction, vents, or cardioplegia to manage make ECMO relatively straightforward when compared to cardiopulmonary bypass in the operating room. A major part of the ECMO Specialist's time is spent recording data hourly on several flow sheets.

The hours required to train someone to become an ECMO Specialist were reported in a recent survey.[13] The average length of didactic instruction is approximately 25 hours and ranged from 12 to 48. A standardized training manual for ECMO Specialists is in preparation by an ELSO committee and should be available soon. ECMO Specialists in training spend many hours in the laboratory actually doing ECMO on animals. Water drills also are used to teach about circuit complications and form the basis of refresher courses for ECMO nurses. No ECMO Specialist is permitted to manage a patient until they have been observed clinically during a preceptorship with either the coordinator or another trained ECMO Specialist. There is a wide range of hours for clinical preceptorships. Some programs have discontinued use of animal laboratory experience, and this may account for the long number of hours spent in some programs to qualify their ECMO Specialists.

Regarding the technical aspects of ECMO, most neonates are cannulated extrathoracically through the right neck vessels. The procedure takes place under sedation. The endotracheal tube is in place, but the ventilator settings are low. In fact the patient can be disconnected from the ventilator for pulmonary lavage or suctioning without worrying about hypoxia because the ECMO circuit is exchanging gas. A variety of monitoring devices, and sometimes chest tubes, are attached to the patient. A bedside nurse is responsible for conventional nursing care just as if the ECMO patient would be a regular ICU patient.

Most neonatal ECMO experience to date has been performed in the veno-arterial (VA) mode. The venous cannula, usually 12 or 14 French, is positioned in the superior vena cava/right atrial junction for removal of venous blood. After passing through the circuit, oxygenated blood is reinfused into the aortic arch via the right common carotid artery. This modality represents a partial bypass, and the heart continues to eject blood. There also is pulmonary blood flow through the entire time, which is another important difference between ECMO and cardiopulmonary bypass. Typically the ECMO pump flow is set to a rate of 100 to 120 cc/kg.

There has been much recent enthusiasm and excellent results with veno-venous (VV) ECMO for neonates. This procedure uses a special single dual-lumen cannula placed in the jugular vein. The major advantage is that the carotid artery is not ligated at the end of the procedure. The major disadvantage is that VV ECMO cannot provide cardiac support. Currently, in about 15% of the cases a VV cannulation must be converted to VA to provide adequate support to the patient.

The typical ECMO circuit is simple: venous blood flows by gravity from the right internal jugular vein to a small venous reservoir mounted in a bladder box that servo-regulates the roller pump in the event of decreased blood volume. Blood then passes through a SciMed membrane oxygenator, a tubular heat exchanger, and then returns back into the right common carotid artery. One-quarter-inch ID tubing is used throughout. The tip of the arterial cannula is positioned just inside the aortic arch. Heparin and fluids are administered into the circuit by volumetric infusion pumps connected before the bladder reservoir. A "bridge" between the arterial and venous lines permits recirculation of extracorporeal blood during priming and trials off ECMO. (Figure 5)

The ECMO circuit is all contained on a stainless steel cart. Because the SciMed membrane is the only FDA-approved oxygenator for long-term use, all ECMO programs currently use it. For the pumphead raceway most programs use the special polyvinyl chloride (PVC) tubing called "Super Tygon." It looks and feels like regular PVC, however it has been formulated for extended use.

Most programs rely on a roller pump, servo-regulated with a bladder box. The purpose of the bladder box is to detect decreased volume on the venous side of the circuit. When this happens, a small silicone rubber bladder collapses, triggering the electric power to be interrupted, and thus stopping the roller pump. Some programs have eliminated the bladder box and rely on pressure transducers for both negative and high positive pressure servo-regulation of the roller pump.[14] Only a few

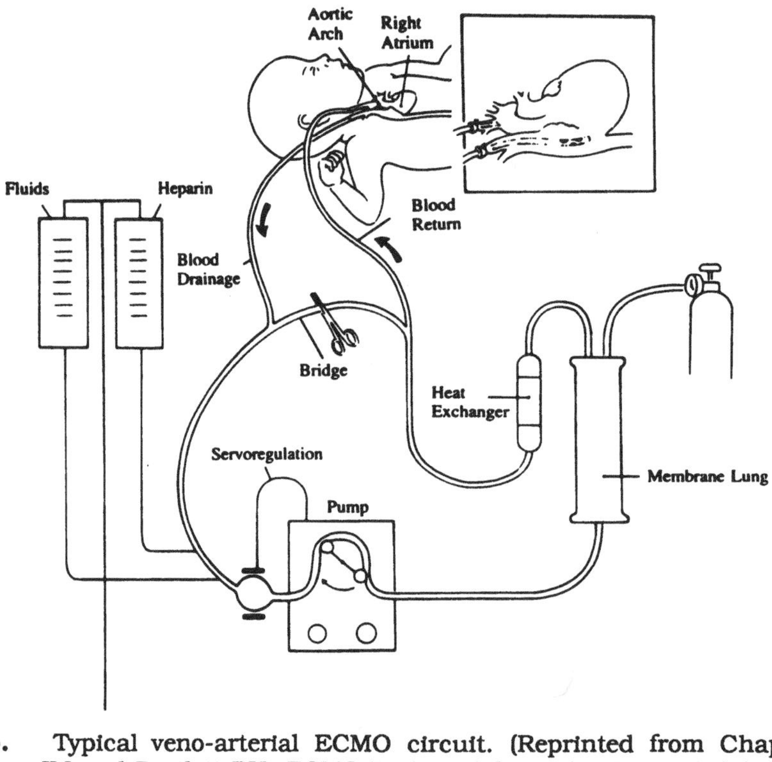

Figure 5. Typical veno-arterial ECMO circuit. (Reprinted from Chapman RA, Toomasian JM and Bartlett RH: *ECMO Technical Specialist Manual*, 9th Ed., 1988, University of Michigan. Used with permission.)

programs use centrifugal pumps for neonates, but they are being used with some frequency in the pediatric or adult patient populations.

Heparin anticoagulation is required during ECMO, just as it is during conventional cardiopulmonary bypass. However, the activated clotting times (ACTs) are typically kept in the 220 to 260 second range, depending on the specific ACT device used for monitoring. Most programs use the Hemochron test with pediatric tubes which require 0.25 cc samples. ACTs are performed every 30 to 60 minutes, and the average dose of heparin is 20 to 50 units/kg/hour by continuous infusion into the circuit.

Regarding monitors, few ECMO teams use an air bubble detector. Of those who do use them, half have the Cobe system which can be used with any manufacturers' pump; we have recently purchased this system and are installing it on the circuit for added protection against air embolism.

In lieu of that approach, the SciMed tubular heat exchanger works quite well as a gross bubble trap with blood entering at the top and exiting the bottom. Neonatal ECMO flows are typically less than 500 cc per minute. We performed a bench top study[15] to quantitate how effective the SciMed heat exchanger was in trapping air bubbles and found that below 400 cc per minute flow no bubbles exited the heat exchanger when challenged with boluses up to 5 cc. However, at higher flows, the heat exchanger does not reliably trap bubbles. Therefore, the move towards performing ECMO in pediatric patients with flows higher than 400 cc per minute has justified the purchase of an air bubble detector in our program.

Other circuit monitors include two pressure displays for continuous measurement of pre and post membrane pressures to detect either a kinked arterial cannula or significant clot formation in the membrane. Another monitoring device is a Doppler to monitor the sound of blood flow through the circuit.[16] If there are any changes in the flow, the ECMO Specialist may detect it immediately. Even more importantly, if any air bubbles pass the sensor a loud clicking noise is heard.

Ventilating oxygen concentration and blood temperature are also monitored to detect problems before they become potentially life-threatening, and an on-line oxygen saturation probe is placed in the venous line to continuously assess tissue perfusion.

WHAT ARE ECMO COMPLICATIONS?

Table 2 lists the most common mechanical complications during more than 5000 neonatal cases. The largest category is classified, "other," and occurs in about 15% of the cases. This reflects the fact that in addition to identifiable components, the entire ECMO circuit is subject to failure including the servo-regulating mechanism, bladder reservoir, gas flow meters or blender, etc.

Clotting remains the most common identifiable complication and it

Table 2. Mechanical complications.

COMPLICATION	INCIDENCE
Clots	9.7 %
Cannula malposition	8.6 %
Oxygenator failure	4.2 %
Air in circuit	2.7 %
Tubing rupture	1.9 %
Other*	14.2 %
ALL	0.41 per pt

Other* refers to non-specified components of ECMO circuit. (Courtesy Extracorporeal Life Support Organization, Ann Arbor, Michigan, July 1991)

occurs in about 10% of the cases. Cannula problems occurred 8.6% of the time. Oxygenator failure occurred 4.2% of the time and is usually manifested by very high inlet pressures due to development of blood clots. Air in the circuit was seen in 2.7% of the cases. Tubing rupture and/or pump failure was seen infrequently. The overall incidence for a mechanical complication is 0.41 per patient. The mean aggregate survival associated with any mechanical complication was 75%, but, of course, causality is not documented nor implied by these data. Obviously, having backup equipment is important in the event a major component in the ECMO circuit fails, and it is specified in the document entitled "Guidelines for Neonatal ECMO Centers" available from ELSO.

To minimize mechanical complications, certain modifications have been used on the circuit in addition to the monitoring previously described. A simple plastic tubing holder can be tucked under the patient's mattress to stabilize the pump lines and cannulae. Using this arrangement it is rare to experience cannula kinking, and we have never had an instance of accidental decannulation which has been reported by others.

To facilitate an oxygenator changeout a double "Y" may be incorporated into the circuit, one before the membrane and one after. In this fashion, one leg can be double-clamped and divided while blood flow to the patient is maintained. The typical time off ECMO support when changing an oxygenator is less than one minute.

Patient complications during ECMO are more numerous than mechanical ones. (Table 3) Intracranial hemorrhage or cerebral infarction occurs in about 15% of the patients. Seizures occur in about 14%, followed by bleeding at the cannulation or surgical site in 13%. Over 10% of the patients require dialysis or hemofiltration. Plasma free hemoglobin values are only modestly elevated in most patients, but serous hemolysis does occur in about 8.6%. The overall incidence for a patient complication is 1.56 per patient, with a 62.6% aggregate survival rate in the patient complication group. While this group appears to fare worse than those experiencing mechanical complications, there are 38 categories of patient complications in the ELSO Registry versus

Table 3. Patient complications.

COMPLICATION	INCIDENCE
Intracranial hemorrhage	15.8 %
Seizures	13.9 %
Bleeding	12.9 %
Dialysis/Hemofiltration	11.6 %
Hemolysis	8.6 %
ALL (38)	1.56 per pt

(Courtesy Extracorporeal Life Support Organization, Ann Arbor, Michigan, July 1991)

13 in the mechanical group which probably accounts for the higher incidence rate in the former.

WHAT IS THE FUTURE OF ECMO?

ECMO is a viable extracorporeal support technique and its use is going to continue to grow in the foreseeable future. As a spin-off, ECMO has promoted better ventilator management techniques in newborns. For example, jet ventilation may not be as damaging as conventional ventilator management with high levels of PEEP. Many centers have not had to put meconium aspiration babies born in-house on ECMO because of an increased awareness of the disease process learned through experience with ECMO.

It also is easy to foresee integration and additional servo-regulation of the ECMO circuit. Most blood loss during ECMO is due to blood sampling for ACTs and other routine laboratory studies. Even when minimal volumes of blood are drawn, the total volume per day approaches 40 to 50 cc, which in a 3 kg infant would account for the entire blood volume after four or five days. Therefore, in-line or on-line monitoring may become an important addition to the ECMO circuit. There has been criticism of VA ECMO because of the necessity to ligate the right carotid artery afterwards. Some groups have surgically repaired the artery, but stenosis rates are high. Veno-venous ECMO with a dual-lumen catheter appears to work very well and there is a tendency to move toward this mode of neonatal ECMO.

Heparin-coated circuits have been advocated and promised for some time, but now truly are becoming available. Trials with the new Medtronic Minimax hollow fiber membrane oxygenator have been performed at a few centers. Of course, heparin-coating the SciMed membrane would be an advantage, and this development appears likely in the near future.

Finally, trials are underway at a few centers with the intravascular oxygenator, or IVOX, which technically is simpler than ECMO.[17] This device may be ideal in carefully selected adults who need assisted ventilation. It is analogous to the intra-aortic balloon pump for cardiac assistance insofar as the IVOX can only provide partial respiratory support. Extracorporeal CO_2 removal is another form of ECMO which has been used with much success in Europe and may offer promise in those adults who need more than an IVOX.

In closing, ECMO represents an exciting outlet for perfusionist involvement. It is likely that experience with patient populations other than neonates will expand. ECMO is becoming a clearly established modality for the postoperative pediatric cardiac patient requiring temporary circulatory support.[18] Improvements in current technique and devices will occur and can be aided by perfusionist input.

ACKNOWLEDGEMENT

The cooperation of Sandy M. Snedecor and the Extracorporeal Life Support Organization (ELSO), Ann Arbor, Michigan in supplying ELSO statistics used in this chapter is gratefully acknowledged; ELSO is supported in part by a grant from the William Randolph Hearst Foundation. Donna F. Graves, R.N. and Jill Chernin, R.N. reviewed the manuscript.

REFERENCES

1. S.C. Faulkner: Letters to the Editor. *Perfusion Life* 8:33; 1991.
2. R.H. Bartlett, A.B. Gazzaniga: Extracorporeal circulation for cardiopulmonary failure. *Curr Problems Surg* 15:1-96;1978.
3. R.H. Bartlett: Extracorporeal life support for cardiopulmonary failure. *Curr Problems Surg* 27:623-705;1990.
4. J.M. Sinard, R.H. Bartlett: Extracorporeal membrane oxygenation (ECMO). Prolonged bedside cardiopulmonary bypass. *Perfusion* 5:239-249;1990.
5. R.A. Chapman, J.M. Toomasian, R.H. Bartlett: *ECMO Technical Specialist Manual.* 9th Edition, Ann Arbor, MI, University of Michigan, 1988.
6. W.J. Rashkind, A. Freeman, D. Klein, R.Q. Toft: Evaluation of a disposable plastic, low volume, pumpless oxygenator as a lung substitute. *J Pediatr* 66:94-102;1965.
7. J.D. Hill, T.G. O'Brien, J.J. Murray, L. Dontigny *et al.*: Prolonged extracorporeal oxygenation for acute post-traumatic respiratory failure (shock-lung syndrome). *N Engl J Med* 286:629-634;1972.
8. R.H. Bartlett, A.B. Gazzaniga, M.R. Jefferies, R.F. Huxtable *et al.*: Extracorporeal membrane oxygenation (ECMO) cardiopulmonary support in infancy. *Trans Am Soc Artif Intern Org* 22:80-93; 1976.
9. W.M. Zapol, M.T. Snider, J.D. Hill, R.J. Fallat *et al.*: Extracorporeal membrane oxygenation in severe acute respiratory failure; A randomized prospective study. *JAMA* 242:2193-2196;1979.
10. J.B. Zwischenberger, R. Bartlett: Extracorporeal circulation for respiratory or cardiac failure. In: *Critical Care*, Edited by Civetta JM, Taylor RW and Kirby RR, Philadelphia: JB Lippincott Co., 144;1629-1637;1988.
11. J.M. Toomasian, R.H. Bartlett: Logistical considerations for establishing an ECMO program. *Proc Am Acad Cardiovasc Perfusion* 5:135-137;1983.
12. R.M. Odell, R. Erickson, R.M. McEwan: Identification of ECMO Specialists and ECMO team composition by profession: Results of a national survey of

ELSO centers, May 1991. Extracorporeal Life Support Organization, 3rd Annual Meeting, (Abstract) p 50;Sept 1991.

13. P.L. Allison, M. Kurusz, D.F. Graves, J.B. Zwischenberger: Devices and monitoring during neonatal ECMO: Survey results. *Perfusion* 5:193-201;1990.
14. J.M. Toomasian, R.A. Chapman, M. McCall, C.E. King *et al.*: Servo-regulation for long term perfusion. *Proc Am Acad Cardiovasc Perfusion* 9:114-117;1988.
15. M. Kurusz, C.S. Cox, M. Girouard, M. Griffin *et al.*: Air trapping capability of the SciMed ECMOtherm heat exchanger. Extracorporeal Life Support Organization, 3rd Annual Meeting, (Abstract) p 11-13, Sept 1991.
16. S.C. Faulkner, M. Kurusz, J.B. Zwischenberger, P.L. Allison *et al.*: Doppler monitoring of venous flow during extracorporeal membrane oxygenation: An inexpensive, readily available monitoring device. *Proc Am Acad Cardiovasc Perfusion* 8:165-169; 1987.
17. C.S. Cox, J.B. Zwischenberger, M. Kurusz: Development and current status of a new intracorporeal membrane oxygenator (IVOX). *Perfusion* 6:291-296;1991.
18. R.C. Groom, A.G. Hill, B.F. Akl, E.A. Lefrak *et al.*: Pediatric perfusion survey. *Proc Am Acad Cardiovasc Perfusion* 11:78-84; 1990.

BIOMATERIALS AND THE DEVELOPMENT OF MEMBRANE TECHNOLOGY

Jeffrey P. Sites, B.S., CT, CCP

Cardiovascular and Extracorporeal Technologies
Plymouth, Minnesota

The significance of the role biomaterials play in the extracorporeal circuit are obvious, and as such are only a very small part of the gigantic family of materials used in contact with living tissue. Our understanding of the action of the material upon biological tissues, or the reaction of the tissue to the material, or interaction between the two, is increasingly important in light of the role the perfusionist and physician plays in utilizing artificial materials to replace an organ or organ segment or to provide life support, either with cardiopulmonary bypass, ventricular assist or an artificial heart. The analysis of this extensive subject has been compared to "a blind soul studying an elephant by touch alone."

A small but highly significant segment of this is to look at the increasing success of long-term support without an artificial lung. The technique of cardiopulmonary long-term support is not by any means similar to that of cardiopulmonary bypass: problems related to protection of the patient from the damaging effects of the extracorporeal circuit is of utmost importance. In this direction, I would like to briefly discuss what a biomaterial is, the biomaterial/blood interaction, and the significance of the materials explored and in current use for artificial lungs.

The term *biomaterial* is taken to mean biocompatible artificial material, or more colloquially as a material which does not cause an adverse reaction in contact with tissue. In heart-lung bypass, we are predominantly worried about blood as a tissue, and its interactions with the foreign materials.

The term *blood compatibility* should be used only in a carefully defined context. There are at least two coagulation mechanisms in the blood, one that predominates in arterial blood flow, with high wall

Cardiac Surgery: Current Issues, Edited by A.C. Cernaianu and A.J. DelRossi Plenum Press, New York, 1992

shear rates, and the other which predominates in venous system with low wall shear rate and flows. Few materials have consistently shown good blood compatibility in both distinctly different environments. Further, experiments with materials in different species of animals cause considerable variation in results. Therefore any statement about blood compatibility should include a description of the conditions under which these data are valid.

The conditions within this context include rheological, as well as enzymatic or metabolic factors. Physical parameters include shear, composed of three specific interrelated variables: the force of shear, the rate at which shear occurs and the resistance of the flow system to shear.

By definition *shear force* is a force, or stress, in which the material (fluid) on one side of an interface pushes/pulls/drags on the material (fluid) on the other side of the interface with a force parallel to the interface.

Shear rate is the relative velocities in laminar flow of parallel adjacent layers of a fluid body under shear force. *Shear resistance* is a tangential stress cause by a fluid (viscosity) and taking place along a boundary/interface of a flow in the tangential direction of local motion (shear drag).

As an example, consider the concern of complement activation and the relationship between the two current gas exchange surfaces, i.e. polypropylene and silicone. In general, all materials induce some degree of complement activation, in the presence of blood, depending upon different system conditions.

Three interacting factors control normal hemostasis, or excessive thrombosis. These are: the thromboresistance of the blood contacting surface, the coagulability of the blood, and the presence of smooth, non-turbulent flow.

Deviations from the normal physiological limits of these three related parameters may lead to thrombosis. Clearly, most prosthetic medical devices, and in particular, blood oxygenators violate these principles, requiring aggressive intervention to preclude a reaction. In addition, surfaces are non-endothelialized and thrombogenic. Flow through or around such a device is often marked by turbulence and focal eddies. A combination of these factors may cause local hypercoagulability in the form of platelets or coagulation proteins.

Typically, biomaterials are not thromboresistant. Prevention of thrombus in functional devices has generally been accomplished by a judicious combination of:

1. Use of material with superior thromboresistance, including surface micro-characteristics which may minimize protein activation.

2. Generation of flow regimens (flow characteristics) which enhance "washing" of the surface (kinetic displacement) and minimize

points of stasis by maintaining an average velocity adequate to resist thrombus formation.

3. Alter the blood chemistry with antithrombotic agents such as anticoagulants and antiplatelet agents.

Considerable effort has been put into the latter, that is the use of anti-clotting agents - used in a shotgun approach with systemic dosing. More recently, work has been done with attaching these agents to the material themselves - the concept of coatings. While effective, this has changed the locus to the first segment of the triad mentioned above. A balance of perspective is necessary considering all three factors are still present, as evidenced by our ability to provide full support of a patient without a coated surface, without systemic anticoagulation and with attention to the second point of the triad, maintaining safe rheological conditions.

HISTORICAL PERSPECTIVE TO MEMBRANE OXYGENATOR DEVELOPMENT

The idea of artificial gas exchange was first demonstrated by Hooke in 1667, with a ventilation technique which lead to the advent of mouth-to-mouth resuscitation. The concept of extracorporeal circulation was suggested by LeGallois in 1812,[1] when he perfused decapitated rabbits by blood injection through the carotid arteries, however, he was unable to demonstrate continuous flow or replacement of the heart due to inadequate technology.

In the 1850's, Brown-Sequard obtained red blood, by "whipping" black blood in a colander type device.[2] He demonstrated the necessity of red blood as a perfusate to obtain nervous activity of isolated mammalian heads.

In 1876, Bunge described oxygenated isolated kidney perfusion. Von Schroeder in 1882 developed a bubble oxygenator by bubbling air into the venous blood in an organ perfusion system. Jacobi in 1890 coupled this concept with a bladder pump to provide pulsatile perfusion for organ preservation.[3]

Blood-filming oxygenators were first reported in 1915, with descriptions of stationary and rotating types following shortly.[4] Perhaps one of the most significant events to occur in this century in regards to cardiovascular surgery was the identification, isolation, and purification of heparin from lung tissue by McKean in 1916. The process was reported in full in 1918 by Howell and Holt which lead immediately to its commercialization.[5]

The next general event occurred in 1934, when Debakey reported the development of the roller pump, not for cardiopulmonary bypass, but for rapid blood transfusion.[6] Alexis Carrel, the father of organ transplantation, and Charles Lindbergh developed in 1935 a perfusion system for isolated organ long-term support, successfully applying the concept of near-normothermic perfusion to an isolated organ.[7]

Gibbon[8] in 1937, combined several techniques to successfully provide systemic cardiopulmonary perfusion in animals utilizing a vertical screen oxygenator and a pneumatically driven bladder pump system.

While Gibbon (1954) is accredited with the first successful use of cardiopulmonary bypass, Dennis[9] (1951) was the first to report a total cardiopulmonary bypass procedure in a 6 year-old girl with an endocardial cushion defect, using a rotating screen oxygenator achieving 40 minutes of bypass time. The patient died from the complexity of the cardiac defect.

Dogliotti[10] (1952) first applied a pump oxygenator version to a human, performing right heart bypass for a mediastinal tumor resection. Ironically, both of these techniques utilized a simple silicone compound developed by Leland Clark[11] in 1950, now known as Antifoam A.

In 1954 Gibbon[12] reported a successful repair of a secundum atrial septal defect (ASD) in an 18 year old girl, utilizing a variation of the screen oxygenator he employed several years earlier, and incorporating Debakey's roller pumps.

In 1955, DeWall[13] introduced a simple helical reservoir and bubble oxygenator. Dr. Lillehei[14] and associates presented the concept of cross-circulation, principally using an adult as the oxygenator and venous reservoir to perfuse an offspring.

The use of membranes in gas exchange devices parallels that of the history of biomedical polymers. The first use of a celluloid polymer was in 1894, when Frankel applied this structured cellulose material to plug holes in the cranium. Ironically this was within a year of the first reported successful operation on a ventricular wound.

Membrane oxygenators were described by Willem Kolff,[15] while in the Netherlands, during the 1920's. Having pioneered the use of structured cellulose, the predecessor of cuprophane, for ion exchange mediums in the process of hemodialysis, he began to recognize that gas, primarily oxygen, could also cross the membrane boundary.

In 1956, Kolff[16] reported a prototype of an untreated polyethylene membrane module as a departure from natural cellulose, recognizing the ease of production and reproducibility. However, he did successfully develop a clinical version of the celluloid coil oxygenator. Also in 1956, Clowes[17] developed a polyethylene plate type membrane oxygenator. The advantage to the Clowes device was that the structure allowed for manipulation of gas transfer gradients both statically (with vacuum) and dynamically (with pressure).[(17)]

At that time, the move toward the utilization of untreated membrane technology was limited by two factors: gas transfer efficiency, through diffusion of oxygen and carbon dioxide across the material, and the size related to volume and surface area. Gas transfer in the

Thickness (um)	Material	O_2	CO_2
75	Cellophane	6	130
20	Polyethylene	8	30
12	Teflon	50	130
25	COPOLYMER (silicone & polycarbonate)	330	1,600
25	Silicone	1,200	6,000

Trade Off: Adequate CO_2 Transfer with Sufficient O_2 Delivery

Figure 1. Relative permeabilities of gas transfer applications. Units are ml/min/m^2. Thickness (μm) refers to the "reference membrane" thickness.

membrane lung is influenced by the solubility of the gas in the mem brane and the gas tension gradient.

These are the same factors as for the native lung. The lung tissue is a diffusion-based gas transfer material as we have described here. The construction of alveolar tissue is a solid membrane over a "leaky" basement material. In a membrane oxygenator, oxygen transfer gradients are typically 5 to 6 times greater than carbon dioxide gradients. Therefore, to provide equal gas exchange, the membrane should be at least 5 to 6 times more permeable to carbon dioxide than to oxygen. A comparison of the non-microporous gas exchange interface biomaterials investigated through the years have demonstrated material limitation for it's application in a blood oxygenator.

CURRENT MATERIALS: POLYPROPYLENE AND SILICONE

Polypropylene and silicone are the two common biomaterials used in today's membrane oxygenators. Polypropylene belongs in the same chemical family as polyethylene. They are one of the lightest of plastics, with significant inertness to most alcohols, soap solutions and synthetic detergents, all of which are part of the interim steps in applying coatings. However, polypropylenes are susceptible to swelling and softening when in the presence of halogenated hydrocarbons and strong oxidizers, while in the presence of water and aliphatic agents (medium molecular weight fats and oils) (Figure 3).

As revealed by the results in Figure 1, polyethylene/polypropylene in itself is a considerably poor gas transfer medium, however it's polymolecular structure and chemical nature make it highly manufacturable and modifiable for many applications.

To enhance gas transfer, the polypropylene material is made microporous most commonly through a stress induction process. Stress induction, simply described in lay terms, refers to a process which induces strain on the weaker bonds *between* molecular chains of a polymer as opposed to those *within* the polymolecular structure. These bonds are separated by force, within a highly controlled process, to create micropores of a given size (Figure 2). Chemical degradation processes have been described for this, but early attempts to incorpo-

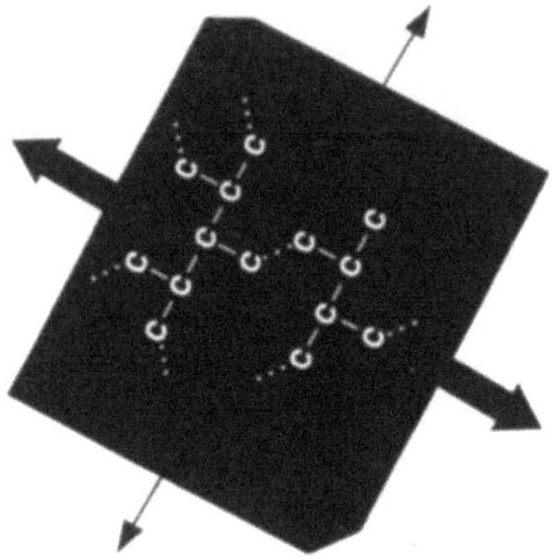

Figure 2. Representation of the vector forces in the stress induction of micropores in polypropylene as used in gas transfer devices.

rate such processed materials into gas exchange devices demonstrated inconsistent gas transfer when used clinically.

Microporous devices are made of expanded materials which substantially alter the chemical structure of the surface, and opens gas channels through which direct gas/plasma interfaces or boundaries are formed. This returns the gas transfer restriction as noted above to the thickness of the plasma boundary layers. However, there is a significant trade off here, i.e., the loss of the hydrophobic nature of polypropylene, causing a high degree of *water flux*, and as such protein denaturation at the pore site.

Silicones, particularly dimethylsiloxane, are other predominant

1. Light
2. Significant Inertness to Soaps, Alcohols, Detergents
3. Electrostatically Neutral
4. Highly Manufacturable
5. Hydrophobic - No Water Flux
6. Susceptible to Swelling and Softening in Presence of Halogenated Hydrocarbons in Presence of Water and Aliphatic Components (medium molecular weight fats and oils)

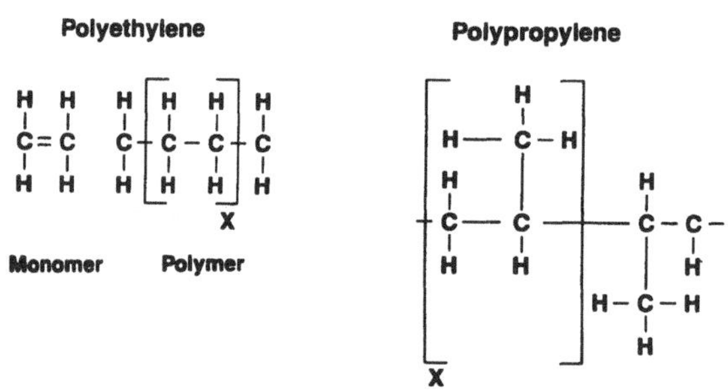

Figure 3. Functional properties and molecular configuration of polyethylene and polypropylene materials.

1. Physiologically Inert
2. Antithrombogenic
3. Non-Toxic Biocompatible/Implant Material
4. Excellent Gas Transfer Media
5. Low Water Flux
6. Non-Microporous Surface
7. No Direct Gas-to-Blood Contact
8. Naturally Electrochemically Negative in Surface Charge - Identical to Normal Blood Vessel Endothelium

Dimethylsiloxane
Silicone Rubber Polymer

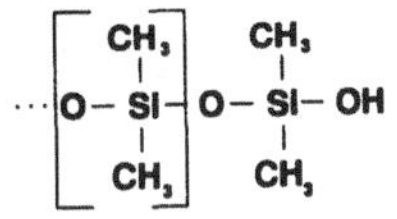

Figure 4. Functional properties and molecular configuration of Dimethylsiloxane.

biomaterials applied in the gas exchange devices. These are semi-organic polymers which have, in certain applications, a high degree of biocompatibility. As shown in the table previously, comparing relative permeabilities, it is highly soluble for oxygen and carbon dioxide. Its limitations are that gas transfer is linearly dependant upon gas tension gradients. Further, as a true rubber-like material, it is very difficult to manufacture. It's primary advantages as a biomaterial are due to it's low water flux as a result of it's hydrophobic nature, as well as it's electrostatically negative surface which leads to a degree of repulsion of similarly charged proteins, whereas polypropylene is electrostatically neutral without modification (Figure 4).

PHYSICAL QUANTITIES INFLUENCING OXYGENATION (GAS TRANSFER)

Gas exchange in the oxygenator can be limited by the plasma boundary layer, gas tension gradient, and dwell time in the gas exchange area. Designs to enhance gas exchange due to some of these engineering restrictions address the blood film thickness, blood path size/geometry, and flows.[18]

An excessive blood film thickness, or plasma boundary layer is counterproductive to efficient gas transfer. Therefore, in light of the dependencies of a microporous device to maintain a plasma boundary layer but not excessively, designs and mode factors to modify the flow path and film thickness have been implemented. The most common technique in a flat sheet device is to use a blood screen which induces secondary flow patterns and also increases dwell time. This concept stems from early work performed by Clowes and Kolff.[16,17]

The diffusion-dependant solid silicone device also needs a minimal plasma boundary layer as any additional thickness decreases diffusion efficiency. The silicone sheet device incorporates a screen within the matrix of the silicone itself which induces secondary flow patterns, a washing effect to minimize plasma layering and increase dwell time. The significant difference between the two types are that, in the silicone membrane, the screen is imbedded and coated, causing a true surface modification; the other being directly in the blood path adding a small amount of surface area for blood contact.

The design of the microporous hollow fiber devices, particularly those with blood flow outside the fibers have inherent blood flow disruption characteristics due to the winding technique, fiber geometry, pore orientation to the flow path, and pressure drop of the device. Under nominal conditions, this creates a predictable environment for the plasma boundary layer.[19]

COATINGS: SURFACE MODIFICATION TO REDUCE THROMBOGENICITY

There is considerable interest in addressing the less than ideal nature of the biomaterials utilized in the membrane oxygenator by "coatings" compounds with the goal of producing surface modification to reduce thrombogenicity.

The concept of coating material to alter its chemical and physical response to blood tissue is not new. The use of silicone as a wetting agent to resist defibrination in the laboratory was described over 100 years ago.[20] Clark's Antifoam A is a surface modification which is applied in every defoamer used today in bubble oxygenators, cardiotomies and hard shell venous reservoirs.

There are two principal approaches to surface modification as it is applied to the extracorporeal circuit. These include the pharmaceutical approach involving antiplatelets and anticoagulant agents, and the use of surfactants, surface active agents, substances. When present in low concentrations in a system, these compounds have the property of adsorbing onto the surfaces or *interfaces* of the system.[20,26]

The development of non-thrombogenic polymers may prevent activation of the thrombogenic mechanism by either tailoring the polymer surface/interface to minimize blood interactions or by selective adsorption. This can be accomplished by incorporating the pharmacologically active agent in the polymer via bulk dispersion or surface immobilization.

BULK DISPERSION: CONTROLLED RELEASE PROCESS

The pharmacologic approach via both bulk dispersion or surface immobilization includes as the predominant agent heparin. The use of heparin in fixed form addresses some problems, depending upon the heparin fraction not bound to the material. Systemic heparinization may induce thrombocytopenia, and prolonged bleeding.

The first application of the process of controlled release heparin was by Gott, in the shunt developed as a vascular bypass.[20,27] He utilized a mediated carbon benzalkonium sulfate treatment.[21] Benzalkonium sulfate (which is a chemical sterilant - or soap) is used to treat the polymer, with a cationic interaction on the surface and anionic interaction in the solvent portion of the treatment media (the wash). Heparin is then exchanged ionically with the sulfate anion, in a second step. This process is currently utilized commercially in two variations on the theme in CPB devices.

The alternative chemical process is to covalently immobilize heparin onto the polymer surface with a complex carbon chain, making it more stable and an overall larger surface. Similar results are achieved in this fashion except that heparin is not as readily exchanged as ionic bonding allows.[22]

Recent reports have also noted that immobilized heparin surfaces adsorb coagulation factors and result in prolonged *in-vitro* clotting times. Most likely this is due to plasma protein interactions with a negatively charged surface.

Platelets may also contact immobilized heparin on the electronegative functional segment of the molecule and inhibit its function. Presumably, this is a time-dependant phenomenon.

Heparin is a drug with many known side effects which are as deleterious to bypass management as they are beneficial. None of the techniques applying a current biomaterial and current surface modification technology will be able to avoid the second of the three problems related to the biomaterial applications in oxygenators, i.e., the flow characteristics.

An advanced process for immobilization of heparin in a gas exchange device has been introduced by Dr. Robert Eberhart[23,24] in Texas, utilizing albumin as opposed to oleic acid chains as the spacer chains to attach the heparin. This process has proved to be successfully applied to most biomaterials and has the distinct advantage of preembedding plasma proteins on the surface, mimicking the endothelialization process in its early stages of biomaterial/tissue contact.

Other agents are being explored as anti-thrombogenic as well as microthrombolytic surface modifiers. Prostaglandins have been applied to many different materials. Prostaglandin I_2, E_2, D_2, are strong stimulants of platelet membrane activity, and are potent inhibitors of platelet adhesion and aggregation.[25] The principal problem identified with using prostaglandins as antithrombotic agents are their ability to be a potent systemic vasodilator. Without accurately controlled release or systemic immobilization the use of these agents could be problematic.

SURFACTANTS

Another area of surface modification being explored is the use of

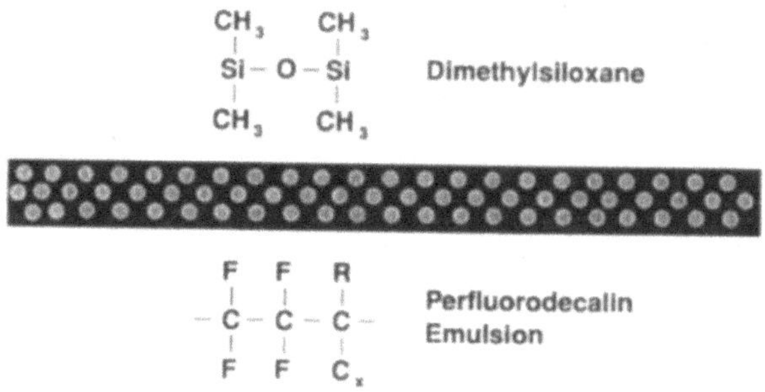

Figure 5. Concept illustraiton of Akagi *et al.* liquid–liquid interface oxygenation (author interpretation).

surfactant-type compounds, which alter phase boundaries on a physical basis, such as siliconizing agents. Surfactants principal function is to lower surface energy potential, lowering work requirements, or *shear* force effects.

However, surfactants typically require a relative steady state. Changes in temperature and physiochemical conditions (electrolyte imbalance, etc.) may result in changes in surfactant activity. Furthermore, the surfactant obviously have a chemical structure amphipathic to the solvent (in this case blood).[25]

The chemical nature of surfactants (*types*) may provide the basis of being incorporated directly into the surface structure of a polymer with fixed, non-biodegradable activity, enhancing the interface phenomena.[26]

In summary, the key to the use of any of the surface modification technologies discussed here, is therefore based upon the *interface phenomenon* within the system (the oxygenator; the entire cardiopulmonary bypass circuit), and the understanding of those phenomena as discussed briefly in the first part of this chapter.

THE FUTURE

Considerable work has been done with developing liquid/liquid interface devices. Akagi and associates[28] reported recently the use of a 3 layer system with low viscosity silicone oil on one layer, and perfluorodecalin, a liquid fluorocarbon, on the other. Blood is circulated in the center layer. The advantages of this system would be the reduction of shear effects, enhanced gas exchange, no water flux or serum leakage, no pressure drag and a "limitless" supply of membrane material, constituted by the liquid-liquid interface (Figure 5).

Closer to current reality, the concept of a hybrid silicone/microporous polypropylene membrane has been explored, and successfully reported in Japan. This material offers ease of manufacturability similar to current techniques, and has enhanced gas transfer with much less protein denaturation and water flux.[29]

A more advanced concept of a hybrid material has been developed by Dillon and Lange[30] of BioMed Sciences which utilizes an interpenetrating polymer network (IPN) incorporating dimethylsiloxane and polytetrafluoroethylene (PTFE, or Teflon). An IPN, or polymer/polymer composite, is defined as a physical blend (as opposed to a chemical blend) of two or more polymers where each polymer forms a network, and each network interpenetrates the other. The biocompatibility, flux rate and gas transfer aspects appear quite promising. Also, it appears to lend itself to manufacturability with current techniques of fabrication for membrane oxygenators.[30]

As a flight of fancy, consider the possibility of the true artificial lung with lung cells cultured in a similar fashion to biotechnology modules for hormone production, as well as artificial livers, which exist today in the laboratory. The degree of biocompatibility of this type of preparation is such that this could lead to a truly implantable artificial lung without the need of immunosuppression. Some of the materials discussed above, in particular the IPN compounds hold great promise in supporting such an application. Further, in light of today's understanding of biocompatibility and immunosuppression, the concept of cross circulation could very well arise again.

As far as the cardiopulmonary bypass, it could also be considered that the oxygenator is really becoming a redundant component. The extracorporeal circuit is intended to give the surgeon a clear and controlled field of operation, which it does. The tradeoff is the risk of hemostatic disruption and blood/tissue effects from the oxygenator. Consideration should be given to cannulation techniques which utilizes the body's natures own oxygenator, i.e. the patient's own lungs. This technique has been applied to more than twenty patients in the United Kingdom utilizing a very simple bypass circuit.[31]

This brief review of the technology available for use every day in our professional activity and it's biointeraction has been discussed. Remember, the strongest force in the universe is the *force of habit*, those habits that simultaneously make us safe practitioners, and also impede our ability to assess differences in technology.

REFERENCES

1. J.J.C. LeGallois: Experiences sur le principe de la vie. Paris, D'Hantel, 1812. Experiments on the principle of life trans. by N.C. and J.C. Nancrede, M. Thomas, Philadelphia, 1813.
2. Brown-Seguard: Recherches experimentales sur les proprietes physiologiques et les usages du sang rouge et du sang noir et leurs principaux elements gayeux, l'oxygene et l'acide carbonique. J Physiol de l'Homme (Paris) 1:95-122,353-367, 729-735;1858.
3. C. Jacoby: Apparat zur Durchblutung isolirter uberlehender Organe. Arch Exp Path (Leipzig) 26:388-400;1890.
4. M. Von Frey, M. Gruber: Untersuchungen uber den Stoffwechel isolierter Organe. Ein Respirations-Apparat fur isolierten Organe *Virchow's Arch Physiol* 9:519-532;1885.

5. W. H. Howell, E.Holt: Two new factors in blood coagulation - heparin and pro-antithrombin. *Am J Physiol* 47:328-41;1918.
6. M.E. DeBakey: A simple continuous flow blood transfusion instrument. *New Orleans Med Surg J* 87:386-389;1934.
7. A. Carrel, C. Lindbergh: The culture of whole organs. *Science* 81:621-623;1935.
8. J.H. Gibbon, M. Gibbon: Artificial maintenance of circulation during experimental occlusion of pulmonary artery. *Arch Surg* 34:1105-1131;1937.
9. C. Dennis, K.E. Karlson, D. Sanderson: Pump oxygenator to support the systemic circulation during the surgical approach of the heart. *Ann Surg* 134:709-721;1951.
10. A.M. Dogliotti: Clinical use of the artificial circulation with a note on intra-arterial transfusion. *Bulletin Johns Hopkins Hosp*:90:131-133;1952.
11. L.C. Clark, Jr., F. Gollan, V. Gopta: Oxygenation of blood by gas dispersion. *Science* III:85-87;1950.
12. J.J. Gibbon, Jr: Application of a mechanical heart and lung apparatus to cardiac surgery. *Minnesota Med* 37:171;1954.
13. R.A. DeWall, C. Whillehen: Design and clinical application of the helix reservoir pump-oxygenator system for extracorporeal circulation. *Post Grad Med* 23:561-573;1958.
14. C.W. Lillehei: Controlled cross circulation for direct vision intracardiac surgery: correction of ventricular septal defects. *Atrioventricularis communis and tetralogy of Fallot.* 17:388-396;1955.
15. W.J. Kolff, H.T.J. Berk: Artificial kidney: dialyzer with great surface area. *Acta Med Seand* 117:121-134;1944.
16. W.J. Kolff, D.B. Effler, L.K. Groves: Disposable membrane oxygenator (heart-lung machine) and it's use in experimental surgery. *Cleveland Clin Qtr* 23:98-114;1956.
17. C.G. Clowes, Jr, A.L. Hopkins, W.E. Nevell: An artificial lung dependant upon diffusion of oxygen and carbon dioxide through plastic membranes. *J Thor Surg* 32:630-37;1956.
18. E.C. Pierce: Membrane oxygenation in cardiopulmonary bypass: Principles and management. Edited by: Taylor, Kenneth; Williams and Wilkins, Baltimore:177-210;1986.
19. J. Scott: *Blood oxygenators, hollow fibers manufacture and applications.* Edited by J. Scott, Noyes Data Corp, NJ:221-228;1981.
20. G.A. Brecher, P.M. Galetti: Materials in extracorporeal circuits, In: *Heart lung bypass: principles and techniques of extracorporeal circulation.* Edited by P.M. Galetti, Grune and Stratton, New York:34-46;1962.
21. S.W. Kim: Heparinized polymers for improving blood compatability. *Med Device and Diagnosis* 6(8):99-103;1984.
22. R. Larsson, D. Larm: Inhibition of thrombin on surfaces coated with immobilized heparin and heparin-like polysaccharides. *Throm Res* 19:43-54;1980.
23. C.C. Tsai, H.H. Huo, P. Kulkarne, R.C. Eberhart: Biocompatible coatings with high albumin affinity. *Trans ASAIO* 36(3):M307-10;1990.
24. J.M. Mrus, R. YN Chao, S.H.Y. Chao, R.C. Eberhart: An extracorporeal perfusion system to bridge pediatric liver transplant candidates. *ASAIO Trans* 36(3):M603-7;1990.
25. Sung W. Kim, C.D. Ebert, T.Y. Lin: Nonthrombogenic polymers - pharmaceutical approaches. *ASAIO Trans* 6(2):76-87;1983.
26. S.L. Cooper, N.A. Peppas: Interfacial phenomena and applications. *Biomaterials, Advances in Chemistry* - Series 199. Edited by: S.L. Cooper, N.A. Peepas. American Chemical Society, NY, 99-135;1982.
27. V.L. Gott, J.D. Whitten: Heparin bonding on colloidal graphite surfaces. *Science* 142:1297-9;1963.

28. H. Akagi, Y. Tanaka, H. Iwata, T. Matsuda, T. Nakatani: A blood-liquid interface for prolonged extracorporeal oxygenation with excellent thrombogenicity. *ASAIO Trans* 36(3):M657-660;1990.
29. Personal communication.
30. M. Dillon, G. Lange: A hybrid interpenetrating network with dimethylsilosane and polytetra fluoroethylene. Company literature, Biomedical Sciences, Inc.
31. L. Cooper: Oxygenator-less bypass. Proceedings of the Third Australasian Society of Extracorporeal Technology Meeting, Auckland, New Zealand, 1990.

THE PHYSIOLOGIC IMPACT OF CARDIAC SURGERY: THE NURSING PERSPECTIVE

Bonnie R. Sakallaris, R.N., MSN, CCRN

Washington Hospital Center
Washington, DC

Cardiac surgery has a profound impact on a patient's physiology. Those who provide care for these patients pre and post operatively must be cognitive of these changes and provide adequate therapeutic interventions. What happens to the patient who enters the operating suite normothermic, anxious, and normotensive? Two to four hours later we care for a comatose, cold, clammy, edematous, hypertensive, tachycardiac patient. This chapter will explore the physiologic impact of cardiac surgery, specifically the areas of hypothermia, cardiopulmonary bypass and from the point of view of the type of surgical procedure.

HYPOTHERMIA

Hypothermia is defined as a decrease in core body temperature of less than 36°C. In the operating room, a patient's core body temperature is lowered to between 21°C and 34°C. This is accomplished through bathing the heart in cooled topical cardioplegia (4°C) and the injection of cardioplegic solution through the aortic root and retrograde perfusion of coronary circulation. Hypothermia is maintained throughout the case by repeated injections of cardioplegic solutions, temperature control on the cardiopulmonary bypass pump, decreased operating room ambient temperature, and anesthesia-induced muscle paralysis.

Hypothermia is an important therapeutic adjunct during cardiac surgery. Hypothermia is based on the Van't Holt effect which predicts a decrease in oxygen consumption (VO_2) which correlates with a decrease in temperature. For example, at 27°C VO_2 is reduced to 50%

and at 17°C VO_2 is only 25% of baseline.[1] The decreased VO_2 provides myocardial protection while the heart is in cardiac arrest during surgery. Aside from it's protective effect, hypothermia has a profound effect on all body systems.

The effects of hypothermia on the cardiovascular system are numerous. Hypothermia is a profound myocardial depressant. The patient's normal cardiac index is correlated to the normal core body temperature. During hypothermia a variety of dysrhythmias may occur. Classically, hypothermia is associated with bradycardia, however,it is not uncommon for the cardiac surgical patient to experience tachycardia as a compensatory mechanism for the low cardiac index due to myocardial depression. In addition, the hypothermic heart is easy and often irritable and ventricular dysrhythmias are not uncommon. Moreover, ventricular dysrhythmias in the hypothermic patient may present problems, since in the hypothermic myocardium is often refractory to cardioversion or defibrillation.[2] During hypothermia, the cardiovascular system presents with a profound increase in pulmonary and systemic vascular resistance. The body attempts to protect vital organs during hypothermia by causing vasoconstriction to the periphery to shunt warmer blood to the core. The vasoconstriction may affect not only peripheral areas but also organ systems such as the kidneys. In addition, blood viscosity increases as temperature decreases, adding to the increased vascular resistance. Cerebral circulation is adversely affected by hypothermia as cerebral blood flow decreases by 7% for each decrease of each °C below normal.[1]

From the cardiovascular perspective, the hypothermic patient can be described as hypertensive with the propensity for developing dysrhythmias such as bradycardia, ventricular ectopy, or tachycardia.

The effects of hypothermia on the pulmonary system include an increase in the anatomic and physiologic dead space. As vasoconstriction occurs in the pulmonary circulation, a lesser number of ventilated alveoli may be participating in gas exchange due to limitation of perfusion. This ventilation/perfusion (V/Q) mismatch produces an increase in dead space. Vasoconstriction also leads to edema of the airways and lung parenchyma. As the patient becomes hypothermic, the normal oxyhemoglobin dissociation relationship is altered, i.e. the oxyhemoglobin dissociation curve shifts to the left. This shift is due to the hemoglobin's increased affinity for oxygen in hypothermic conditions. The patient may present with a normal arterial oxygen saturation (SaO_2), however, with a poor PaO_2. Finally, hypothermia affects CO_2 production. During hypothermia, areas of the body that are poorly perfused begin to experience anaerobic metabolism with increased active acid production. As the patient re-warms, CO_2 production starts to increase in association with increased muscle movement and shivering. During re-warming, the products of anaerobic metabolism coupled with increased CO_2 enter the circulation and cause metabolic acidosis.

From the prospective of the respiratory system, the overall picture is a patient who is hypoxic with a near normal SaO_2 and a metabolic and respiratory acidosis.

Hypothermia produces profound metabolic and biochemical changes. Electrolyte imbalances include hyponatremia and hypocalcemia. Cardiac surgical patients are characterized by profound total body hypokalemia due to an extracellular movement of potassium coupled with enhanced diuresis. During hypothermia, insulin production is suppressed causing a transient hyperglycemia. During re-warming, insulin production resumes and serum glucose levels should return to normal. Progressive metabolic acidosis results from protein catabolism with nitrogen loss, anaerobic metabolism in peripheral tissues, and increased CO_2 production when shivering begins. VO_2 is greatly affected by body temperature. During profound hypothermia, VO_2 is decreased, however, when the patient re-warms VO_2 increases and can reach 200% to 500% of normal as shivering begins.[3]

The net metabolic and biochemical effect of hypothermia results in hypokalemia, hyperglycemia, metabolic acidosis and a profound oxygen deficit.

CLINICAL IMPACT

Since hypothermia acts as a hypnotic, the typical hypothermic patient will appear more anesthetized than a warmer patient. Hypertension, dysrhythmias, and decreased perfusion to the periphery and non-vital organs may be encountered. Patients may experience hypoxia (despite a normal SaO_2) combined with metabolic and respiratory acidosis. The patient may be hypokalemic, hyperglycemic, and demonstrate altered VO_2 (both very low consumption and then very high consumption).

Nursing Interventions

Nursing interventions are aimed at counteracting the adverse effects of hypothermia while rewarming the patient. The rewarming process starts as patients are weaned from cardiopulmonary bypass. The heat exchange unit rewarms the core usually to about 36°C, however, patient's temperature registers at 34 or 35°C on admission to ICU. A phenomenon called "after-drop" (rebound) occurs in the ICU. As warmed core blood mixes with the still cool peripheral blood, after-drop occurs causing a relapse in body temperature. Post operative re-warming is a controversial and much debate has been generated. Studies comparing different types of rewarming interventions using untreated blankets, warmed blankets, electric blankets, and water filled hyperthermia blankets found no difference in time to rewarm. Other therapies such as warmed IV fluids, warmed and humidified respiratory gases, and infrared lights have been also compared to conventional blankets and no difference in rewarming time was found. The only therapies found to decrease warming time were increased operating room ambient temperatures (up to 90°F), and the application of convective warming therapy.[1]

The treatment of the postoperative shivering is also controversial. The first four postoperative hours are most critical for rewarming. Shivering occurs in a sequential manner progressing from masseters to the pectoral muscles, the muscles of the trunk, and then finally the long muscle groups. Shivering increases VO_2 up to 500% of normal, however, this is not an effective postoperative warming mechanism. Shivering can be controlled or stopped with sedation, analgesics, and paralysis.[4] The cost:benefit ratio must be considered in the decision regarding treatment of shivering. Patients who are sedated and paralyzed may take longer to recover from anesthesia and therefore, are intubated and mechanically ventilated for longer time periods. Patients who are allowed to shiver will increase their oxygen demand dramatically. If their left ventricular function is adequate to the demand they may compensate. However, in patients with left ventricular impairment, or inadequate myocardial oxygen supply/demand, the consequences could be hemodynamic instability, or myocardial infarction.

Hypothermia may cause severe vasoconstriction which may be not well tolerated by the cardiac surgical patient. Cardiac index falls as a result of increased afterload, and the graft anastomosis sites may be jeopardized by the high pressures. Vasodilator therapy is commonly utilized to reduce systemic vascular resistance. Agents such as nitroprusside, apresoline, and nitroglycerine are commonly used.

Hypothermia-induced hyperglycemia is not usually treated as the insulin suppression is reversed when the patient warms. The exception would be the diabetic patient in whom insulin production is already impaired.

EFFECTS OF CARDIOPULMONARY BYPASS

Cardiopulmonary bypass (CPB) provides body perfusion during cardiac arrest. During CPB, the operation can be performed on a still, dry surgical field. CPB represents an artificial means to oxygenate and circulate blood. Blood is removed through a cannula in the right atria or double cannulas placed in the inferior and superior vena cava. The heparinized blood runs through circuitry, the membrane oxygenator, and then is returned via the aortic cannula. CPB circulates oxygenated blood at low flow rates, low pressure, in a non-pulsatile manner. During CPB significant alterations in the patient's physiology occur.

CPB results in profound fluid shifts due to an immediate decrease in oncotic pressure. Bypass circuits are primed with 500 to 1000 cc of crystalloid such as lactated Ringer's solution. The volume is given at the beginning of bypass, immediately diluting the intravascular pull and decreasing the oncotic pressure. Blood cells passing through the circuitry and roller pumps may be damaged or destroyed releasing substances which may change the permeability of capillary membranes which are no longer capable of maintaining water and plasma proteins into the vascular space causing leakage into the interstitial spaces. In addition, both low pressure and non-pulsatile flow decrease the hydrostatic pressure, which is part of the normal exchange mechanism from the intravascular to the interstitial space.[5]

The net effect of CPB is a third space syndrome, characterized by an increase in total body water but with a severe intravascular volume deficit. Although this phenomenon is common to all surgical procedures, it is greatly exaggerated when the patient undergoes CPB.

During procedures with CPB, endocrine responses may be triggered by low pressure and non-pulsatile blood flow. Pressure and volume receptors detect hypotension and low volume. Messages are sent to the brain and the endocrine response is initiated, resulting an increase in renin secretion and the activation of the renin-angiotension system. Renin is a potent systemic vasoconstrictor, including the renal artery beds. Antidiuretic hormone (ADH) release has been measured at levels 2000 times than normal.[6] ADH causes water retention and severe vasoconstriction, particularly in the renal artery beds and the coronary arteries. The effects of increased ADH levels are persistent up to 8 hours postoperatively and appear to be greater in the coronary artery bypass grafting (CABG) population than in the valve replacement population. Due to the decrease in intravascular volume, aldosterone is released to maintain sodium and the intravascular water. Aldosterone is also a very potent vasoconstrictor.[6] The overall effects of CPB on the endocrine system may result in severe vasoconstriction and decreased renal blood flow.

During CPB catecholamines production increases to up to 1000 times normal with resultant increase in heart rate and blood pressure.[6] Insulin release may be suppressed with an enhanced glycogenolysis. The overall effect is a hypertensive, tachycardiac, hyperglycemic patient.

Coagulopathy is often encountered in patients undergoing CPB. Systemic heparinization is used for anti-coagulation as blood flows through artificial circuitry. Heparin is usually reversed by protamine. Mechanical destruction of blood cells, particularly platelets, occurs causing disruption in the normal coagulation process with a decrease in platelet function and destruction of coagulation factors. The net result is increased postoperative bleeding.

Pulmonary changes may result from lack of ventilation and perfusion during cardiopulmonary bypass. As the lungs experience minimal ventilation, the alveoli are not expanded enough to stimulate the production of surfactant and atelectasis may result. Lack of perfusion causes sequestration of blood in the pulmonary microcirculation, formation of microthrombi, anoxia, destruction of capillary walls, and the appearance of edema. As ventilation is resumed, atelectasis, and acidosis may occur.

With a usual mean arterial pressure of 40 to 60 mmHg during CPB, cerebral perfusion is greatly affected. Decreased cerebral perfusion is usually tolerated well due to decreased VO_2 but is further compromised in the presence of carotid disease. Emboli formation is a threat to the cerebral circulation throughout CPB and in the postoperative period. Embolic particles may migrate from a left ventricular thrombus, the disruption of an aortic plaque, air in the circuitry, or microemboli in the pulmonary circulation. The literature reports a variety of neurological consequences after CPB, ranging from subtle personality and mood changes to severe cerebral anoxia with permanent structural damage.

Nursing Interventions

Nursing interventions are aimed toward restoring and maintaining hemodynamic stability, and optimal organ perfusion. Volume resuscitation is vital in the postoperative period. Guided by hemodynamic parameters such as a stable blood pressure, adequate pulmonary artery occlusion pressure (PAOC) and central venous pressure (CVP), optimal cardiac index, and adequate urine output, volume resuscitation varies from institution to institution. Generally, colloid or high molecular weight solutions are more employed than crystalloid. Blood products may be required if bleeding complications or oxygen supply problems develop.

Blood pressure management is necessary to optimize cardiac index and to prevent stress on vascular suture lines. Vasodilators such as nitroprusside, and nitroglycerine are utilized.

Adequate ventilation after cardiac surgery is vital as all patients will displace some degree of atelectasis. Usually the patient is ventilated with slightly higher tidal volumes and a PEEP of $5mmH_20$. Arterial oxygen saturation is closely monitored and FiO_2 titrated as needed.

Cerebral perfusion is maintained by avoidance of hypotension. Particular attention should be taken if the patient has a significant history of neurological disease. Renal perfusion is optimized through adequate volume resuscitation and the use of low dose alpha-adrenergic drugs such as dopamine as required.

PROCEDURE SPECIFIC ALTERATIONS

The type of surgery performed will impact the patient's physiology in different ways. For example, some procedures will require more chest retraction than others. Some procedures are performed for chronic rather than acute pathology. Some surgeries require manipulation of the lung parenchyma. The specific procedure must be taken into consideration when planning for nursing care.

SAPHENOUS VEIN GRAFTING VS INTERNAL MAMMARY ARTERY GRAFTING

Saphenous vein grafting (SVG) differs from internal mammary artery (IMA) grafting in several important ways. For example, IMA procedures are associated with increased respiratory complications, bleeding, and pain. IMA procedures require more chest retraction and dissection than SVG, and necessitates the invasion of the pleural space with manipulation of lung parenchyma. IMA demonstrate slightly less flow initially than SV as arteries are less distensible than veins. There is still controversy as to whether patients undergoing IMA grafting have greater infection rates than those undergoing SVG. The only positive association with increased infection rates is proven in diabetic patients undergoing bilateral IMA grafting. IMA grafting presents better long-term patency rate than SVG. Approximately 70-80% of all IMA grafts are patent at 10 years. SVG carrying a 70% restenosis rate at 7 years.[7] The long-term benefits of each type of procedure should be put in balance when the operative decision making process takes place.

VALVE REPLACEMENT

Valve replacement and repair procedures are often associated with conduction problems, particularly atrio-ventricular blocks. As the cardiac valves surround the AV node and the Hiss bundle, conduction defects occur due to swelling and irritation of this area or due to the pressure of suture lines through the conduction structures. Valvular disease is usually associated with chronic heart changes. Dilated or hypertrophic ventricles will maintain after valve replacement or repair.[8] Hemodynamic assessment must be performed in light of these chronic changes. The presence of mechanical valves necessitate anticoagulation when clinically possible. The patient will eventually require prophylactic antibiotics and anticoagulation for life.

ALTERNATIVE CONDUITS

With the increase in redo bypass procedures, the use of alternative conduits such as the gastro-epiploic artery, the inferior epigastric artery, and alternate venous conduits has become necessary. Each of these conduits requires increased dissection to harvest. The use of gastro-epiploic arteries may be associated with an increased incidence of ileus, pain, and infection. Each of these procedures may increase the operative time and therefore, the complications associated with prolonged surgery.

Nursing Interventions

Each procedure is associated with specific pathophysiology which must be considered when planning nursing interventions. Increased bleeding, conduction defects, and vasospasm may occur. The surgery may have been prolonged and involved the abdomen as well as the chest. Each patient will present a different clinical picture depending on the procedure involved. Nursing interventions are planned to prevent complications associated with each procedure. Nitroglycerine is often utilized at low doses to prevent vasospasm. If the conduit is small, or EKG changes are noted, higher dose nitroglycerine may be necessary for arterial dilatation. Coagulopathies and associated bleeding are treated with coagulation factor replacement, lowered MAP, and higher PEEP. Pulmonary complications associated with CABG are prevented by maintenance of chest tubes, and adjustment of ventilation with appropriate tidal volumes and PEEP. Patients who have undergone valve surgery may have pacer wires. Anticoagulation started after chest tubes removal should be monitored for the life of the mechanical valve. When an alternative conduit has been utilized such as the gastro-epiploic, care should be given to prevent ileus, infection and increased medication for pain should be anticipated.

This chapter has analyzed the many causes of the postoperative problems that we deal with every day as we care for the patient after cardiac surgery. To summarize, while the patient is in the operating room they experience profound hypothermia, low pressure, non-pulsatile blood flow. They are subjected to manipulation of their homeostasis, and surgical restructuring. All of these factors combine to cause profound physiologic impact which must be considered in our planning of nursing care.

REFERENCES

1. D.D. Feroe, S.D. Augustine: Hypothermia in the PACU. *Critical Care Clinics of North America* 3(1),135-144;1991.
2. C. Biddle: Hypothermia: Implications for the critical care nurse. *Critical Care Nurse*, 5(2):34-37;1985.
3. R. Phillips, P. Skov: Rewarming and cardiac surgery: A review. *Heart & Lung* 17:511-520;1988.
4. S.K. Oliver, E. Fuessel: Control of postoperative hypothermia in cardiovascular surgery patients. *Critical Care Nursing Quarterly* 12(4):63-68;1990.
5. A.J. Ley: Fluid therapy following intracardiac operation. *Critical Care Nurse* 8(1):26-35;1988.
6. A.P. Weiland, W.E. Walker: Physiologic principles and clinical sequelae of cardiopulmonary bypass. *Heart & Lung* 15(1):34-39;1986.
7. L.S. Kern: Advances in the surgical treatment of coronary artery disease. *J Cardiovasc Nurs* 1:1-14;1986.
8. L.H. Schakenbach: Physiologic dynamics of acquired heart disease. *J Cardiovasc Nurs* 1:1-17;1987.

THE AUTOMATIC IMPLANTABLE CARDIOVERTER DEFIBRILLATOR; SURGICAL CONSIDERATIONS AND PRE- AND POSTOPERATIVE NURSING CARE

Rosemary Volosin, R.N., MSN

Department of Surgery
Division of Cardiothoracic Surgery
University of Medicine and Dentistry of New Jersey
Cooper Hospital/University Medical Center
Camden, New Jersey

Approximately a half million people die suddenly every year in the United States. In most cases, a malignant ventricular tachyarrhythmia is the final common pathway making this a major unresolved health problem in the United States today. About 20-30% will survive their arrest, however, the recurrence of sudden cardiac death at one year is about 30%. In patients with recurrent, sustained ventricular tachycardia or syncope of unknown origin, the recurrence is about 40% at one year. While the majority of patients who have a cardiac arrest have coronary artery disease, only about 20% present with an acute myocardia infarction (MI) at the time of their arrest.[1] Most commonly, these patients have a history of MI in the past which creates myocardial scarring, thereby providing a substraight for abnormal electrical conduction, making them prime candidates for these types of arrhythmias.

Treatment alternatives for these patients consists of drug therapy, device therapy or surgical oblation. The problem is the decision making process of which type of therapy is best for each patient. While there have been additions and recent deletions of antiarrhythmics on the market, there are several problems with antiarrhythmic therapy. One problem is that of proarrhythmia which can occur in about 15% of the patients who are discharged on antiarrhythmic medication. There is not total agreement at this time on what exactly is the definition of proarrhythmia, why it occurs, or who gets it, but it most likely has to do with both the chemical makeup of the drug and the actual physiopathology of arrhythmias. Another problem with drugs is that they are expensive, making patient compliance difficult. They also have many

Cardiac Surgery: Current Issues, Edited by A.C. Cernaianu and A.J. DelRossi Plenum Press, New York, 1992

side effects which can cause drug intolerance in certain patients. Lastly, the substrate for arrhythmias may change over time, making an initially effective drug, no longer effective for that patient.

Surgical therapy such as endocardial resection, aneurysmectomy and cryoablation are effective for a specific population of patients. When a patient is a candidate for this type of therapy, success is 80-90%. It works best in patients whose arrhythmias are mappable. Using endocardial mapping techniques to find and isolate the area of the myocardium from which the arrhythmia arises, it can then be surgically removed.

An alternative of therapy for these patients is the implantation an automatic implantable cardioverter (AICD) therapy. Currently on the market is the AICD defibrillator which is manufactured by Cardiac Pacemakers, Incorporated (CPI), Minneapolis, Minnesota. This chapter will mainly concentrate on the AICD because it is the device which is currently available on the market. However, more implantable cardioverter defibrillators (ICDs) will be appearing on the market in the near future. This chapter will focus on the device work, the current devices on the market, future devices, surgical techniques and then pre and postoperative nursing care of patients in whom such a device has been implanted.

The AICD was invented in 1966 by Dr. Michelle Mirowski from Johns Hopkins University. She came up with the idea for an implantable cardioverter defibrillator as a therapy for sudden cardiac death victims. However, the first animal implant was not performed until 1975. The first human implant took place in 1980. In 1982 cardioverting capabilities were added to the device. FDA approval was obtained in 1985. In 1988 the first programmable device was introduced. This represented a big breakthrough because prior devices had fixed rates and circuitry. Now these programmable devices allow us to tailor the device for any particular needs the patient might develop. In 1990 there were 10,000 implants and by 1991 over 15,000 implants in the United States.

CURRENT INDICATIONS FOR AICD IMPLANTATION

Current indication for the implantation of the AICD are: Treatment of ventricular tachycardia and ventricular fibrillation in patients at high risk for sudden cardiac death. AICD is also indicated for patients who survived one episode of a cardiac arrest presumably due to unstable ventricular tachycardia/ventricular fibrillation not associated with an acute myocardial infarction. In the absence of a cardiac arrest, in patients with recurrent ventricular tachycardia and inducible sustained ventricular tachycardia or fibrillation, with hypotension despite conventional antiarrhythmic drug therapy.

THE COMPONENTS OF THE AICD

The AICD consists of a pulse generator which is powered by a lithium battery, housed in a titanium case with an epoxy head where the leads are plugged in. It weighs about a half pound and has a monitoring life of 3-5 years. There is also an apical patch lead, either large or small. These are the more morphology sensing leads which deliver the defibrillatory shock to the heart. It also can be used as what is called a superior vena cava (SVC) lead which acts in the same manner. In the case where patches were used during an implant, the shock goes from patch to patch. In the case where an SVC lead is used, the shock goes from SVC lead to patch. There are also two epicardial rate sensing leads which sense when the heart is in ventricular tachycardia and sends a message to the generator to begin to charge and deliver the defibrillatory shock. The patch leads are sutured to the myocardium at the time of implantation. The epicardial sensing leads are screwed onto the surface of the myocardium.

A new system for implanting these devices is call the Endotak. It is manufactured by CPI, but newer devices coming out on the market from other companies may use this type of system. It consists of a transvenous, right ventricular bipolar sensing lead which has a distal spring on the end which sits in the right ventricle and a proximal spring which lies in the superior vena cava or the right atrium. The polarity of the distal and proximal spring leads can be reversed. The defibrillatory shock can be delivered between the distal and proximal lead, however, if this does not work, a submuscular patch may also be used in conjunction with the lead in order to achieve defibrillation. The Endotak has been submitted to the FDA in December 1991 and approval may be granted in 1992.

The defibrillator works by monitoring heart activity and treats ventricular tachycardia or ventricular fibrillation by delivering direct, current counter shock to the heart through the implanted system. The way the CPI VenTak P device works is that it has two direct detection parameters, rate and probability density function (PDF)which must be met before the device will charge and shock. Rate is a simple concept. To fulfill the rate parameter, the patient's heart rate must exceed the rate cutoff of the device which is a programmable feature. For instance, if the rate cut off is 155, the ventricular tachycardia rate must exceed 155 before the device will charge and shock. The rate range on the device is 120-200 beats per minute. Ideally, the rate cutoff should be less than the patient's ventricular tachycardia rate, but greater than the maximum sinus rate.

The second parameter, PDF, is based on the electrogram morphology, or what the rhythm looks like. In sinus rhythm, the electrogram spends more time at baseline than in ventricular tachycardia or ventricular fibrillation. PDF is a measurement of relative time on the baseline. The PDF is a parameter which can be turned off and rate only can be used for ventricular tachycardia or ventricular fibrillation detection. The device will deliver it's first shock within 10-35 seconds after sensing ventricular tachycardia or ventricular fibrillation. The amount of energy delivered on the first shock is programmable from 0.1 joules on up to 30 joules. If the first shock successfully converts the rhythm, the device returns to monitoring function. If not, it will charge and shock again at 30 joules. The device will deliver up to 5 shocks and then it must see 35 seconds of a normal rhythm before it will reset to shock again. Therefore, when planting these devices,it is very important to determine the defibrillation thresholds in the operating room.

The most common surgical approach used for implanting the system is the median sternotomy. This approach is used with concomitant surgery such as coronary artery bypass grafting. Also, lateral thoracotomy and more recently the subxiphoid approach are gaining popularity. The surgical implant sequence consists of an initial checkout of the equipment and then the implantation of the system and evaluation of the lead signals. The patches and epicardial leads are implanted and then tested for the ability to convert ventricular fibrillation or ventricular tachycardia. The patch leads may be moved a number of times on the surface of the myocardium to achieve the best defibrillation threshold. The implant pocket is constructed and the leads are tunneled through to the abdomen where they are connected to the AICD and conversion testing is performed. The device is then implanted, activated and tested for the ability to convert ventricular tachycardia and ventricular fibrillation. Once the AICD is implanted it is isolated and retested and satisfactory signals and defibrillation thresholds are obtained and the pulse generator is implanted and the incision is closed.

Possible surgical complications include thrombosis, atelectasis or pneumonia, seroma or hematoma at the generator site, pneumothorax, symptomatic pleural effusion or infection. Possible complications involving the pulse generator include pocket infection, lead fracture and failure to terminate ventricular tachycardia or ventricular fibrillation. Complication rate overall for the AICD implantation is less than 1%.[2]

AICD patient's management involves addressing the psychosocial issues associated with receiving the device, extensive patient education and the management of the postoperative implant care. Of course, the type of post implant care depends on the surgical approach which is used.

Standard nursing measures involve monitoring vital signs, chest tube drainage, assessing respiratory status and breath sounds, arterial blood gases, encouraging the patient to promote cough and deep breath after extubation, assessing bleeding at the incision sites. It is also important to watch for signs of infection and remember to mobilize the patient early and give pain medication when doing so and also to offer emotional support when necessary.[3] It is also important to assess for factors that may predispose the patient to arrhythmias either atrial or ventricular, such as electrolyte imbalance, hypoxia, ischemia or concomitant medications.

Post implant, the patient will probably be in the intensive care unit. It is important thing to know if the device is activated or deactivated and to know if the device is on or off at all times and know the rate cutoff, to be knowledgeable of the activation and deactivation procedures. The device is activated and deactivated with a donut magnet which can be applied directly to the surface of the abdomen over the device for 30 seconds. A continuous tone of thirty seconds means that the device is off. After 30 seconds it will beep synchronously with the heart rate indicating that the device is now activated. If a device is active it will charge and shock for rhythms that meet the rate criteria. This includes atrial fibrillation with a rapid ventricular response or non-sustained ventricular tachycardia. Therefore, one of the most important points is to know if the device is on or off and what will it charge and shock for. If a device is off, there will be no time to turn the device on using a magnet before the patient becomes hemodynamically unstable. Therefore, it will be necessary to defibrillate the patient externally using an external defibrillator. The device is not influenced by external defibrillation. Education of the patient should be performed preimplant, predischarge and during the follow-up.

Preoperatively, it is important to reinforce the explanation on the AICD principle and it's application to the patient's condition, and provide the patient with an instruction manual to facilitate questions and answers, allow sufficient time for questions and feedback and reinforce the explanation regarding the surgical procedure. Prior to discharge, the patient must be informed to avoid strong magnetic fields which can inadvertently deactivate the device. The patient should avoid wearing restrictive clothing. Reviewing the CPI patient manual before discharge is of utmost importance. Discussing signs of infection at the implant and reviewing the physician's recommendations is also important.

Follow-up education consists of reviewing the importance of regular visits to the outpatient office. The follow-up tests in the office provide information on device function and insure proper operation. Also the patient should notify the physician if they are planning an extended vacation or if they are moving. It is important to address the psychosocial issues involved with receiving an AICD. Patients may be anxious about having an implanted device, receiving surgery or shocks. Depression related to the illness, and a long history of hospitalization may be encountered. The families of these patients are dealing with a potential loss of a loved one. They may be concerned about the tests, the operative procedure, the need for the implanted device or may express their anxiety in a number of ways, for example, by overprotecting the patient. It is important to assist the patient and the family by providing pre - and postoperative implant education. A psychosocial and occupational history should be obtained on all patients to determine if counseling is warranted. Emotional support can be provided through such things as support groups. It may also be helpful to bring a patient into the hospital who already has an AICD implanted, to talk with the patient who is receiving the AICD to help them to see what life with an AICD is like. Overall, these patients can do very well with proper follow-up and emotional support when necessary. They go on to lead happy and productive lives, travel and pursue the activities which they enjoyed prior to receiving the device.

REFERENCES

1. L.N. Horowitz, A.H. Harken, J.A. Kastor, et al: Ventricular resection guided by epicardial mapping for the treatment of recurrent ventricular tachycardia. *N Eng J Med* 302:591;1980.
2. S.A. Moser, D. Crawford, A. Thomas: Caring for patients with implantable cardioverter defibrillators. *Crit Care Nurse* 8(2):52-65;1988.
3. D.K. Cooper, B.K. Valladares, L.G. Futterman: Care of the patient with the AICD: A guide for nurses. *Heart and Lung* 16(6)Part 1:640-648;1987.

THORACIC TRAUMA AND TRAUMATIC RUPTURE OF THE DIAPHRAGM

Joan Perks, R.N., M.S.N., C.E.N.

Manager of Emergency Services
Atlantic City Medical Center
Atlantic City, NJ

The preoperative diagnosis of a traumatic diaphragmatic rupture is difficult. Frequently, this injury may be overlooked because of the severity of other organ system dysfunctions upon presentation. The importance of assessment of the trauma patient and the epidemiology of this entity will be presented in this chapter with emphasis on components of a primary and secondary survey.

Diaphragmatic rupture results from severe blunt trauma to the lower chest or abdomen, and is most commonly a result of motor vehicle accidents. It may also result from other types of crushing injuries, such as a fall of a great height, or from blows by an object to the lower chest or the abdomen. It is believed that the incidence of diaphragmatic rupture is increasing and it appears to parallel the increase of the rise in motor vehicle accidents.

Since the severity of the traumatic rupture varies, the true incidence of traumatic rupture of the diaphragm is not really known. The site for herniation of abdominal viscera, incarceration, obstruction, or strangulation may follow any trauma or diaphragmatic rupture. For this reason, it is important to identify and to repair penetrating injuries to the diaphragm. Blunt disruption to the diaphragm occurs when forces are so severe, that they are dissipated throughout the abdomen and abdominal cavity, forcing the abdominal viscera into the chest and perhaps rupturing one of the leaflets of the diaphragm.

With the increased sophistication of management in the field, inpatient caretakers must take a look at both the advantages, and the limitations of those that are treating and assessing individuals in the field. Field management is generally comprised of a primary survey and a secondary survey. The primary survey includes evaluating the air-

Cardiac Surgery: Current Issues, Edited by A.C. Cernaianu and A.J. DelRossi Plenum Press, New York, 1992

way, cervical spine control, and evaluation of initial level of consciousness. It comprises the assessment of the circulation, and bleeding. The secondary survey, and the pre-hospital scene assesses vital signs, attempts to take a history of the patient's traumatic event, head to toe physical examination (including neurological) followed by bandaging and splinting with continued monitoring.

A high index of suspicion for diaphragmatic rupture should be raised during the primary and the secondary evaluation in the field and then relate that information to the mechanism of injury. The diaphragm is a dome shaped muscular organ attached posteriorly to the first, second, and third lumbar vertebrae, anteriorly to the lower sternum, and laterally to the costal margins dividing the thoracic and abdominal regions. There are three openings. The aorta passes through at the T-12 level, the esophagus passes through the opening at T-10, and the vena cava passes through the opening at T-8. The phrenic nerve which innervates the diaphragm, passes through the thorax along the posterior lateral aspect of the pericardium on both sides and divides into the anterior and posterior branch. The diaphragm is important in respiration along with intercostal musculature. It is considered the primary muscle involved in respiration. The diaphragm's semispheric shape, with it's concave surface facing the abdominal cavity, and it's convex surface facing the thoracic cavity, allows it to increase the volume of the thoracic cavity with contraction, and decrease the volume with it's relaxation. Depending on the size of the rupture or the location, the diaphragmatic rupture may remain asymptomatic for a long period of time post injury. This may even be discovered by other healthcare workers, i.e. nurses or physicians in the trauma medical-surgical units, or even upon admission and stay in a trauma rehabilitation center.

When symptoms appear, they are mainly related to the herniation of the abdominal content into the chest. This is problematic because of the displacement of the pleural space. Symptoms that patients would exhibit with a diaphragmatic rupture would be chest pain, orthopnea, or dyspnea. Referred diaphragmatic pain may also be located in the scapular area. Severe dyspnea is generally related to a very progressive, gastric distention due to an obstruction, or to the stomach protruding through the diaphragm. Approximately half of these injuries are discovered during exploration of intra-abdominal injury. It has been suggested that diagnostic tests be more widely used in assessing for this type of injury. Tests suggested in the early recognition of diaphragmatic injuries include thoracoscopy, ultrasound, CAT scan, liver-spleen scan, and contrast gastrointestinal studies. However, most commonly, a diaphragmatic rupture confirmation is made from a chest roentgenogram. The algorithm for diagnosis and management of penetrating injury of the chest or upper abdomen is quite simple. When immediate surgery is needed, the patient is taken to the operating room where careful examination of both hemidiaphragms are examined. When injury is present, immediate repair is done. When urgent surgery is not required, the patient undergoes a chest x-ray, and when the diaphragmatic silhouette is abnormal, a nasogastric tube should be placed. At that point in time, different tests, such as liver-spleen scan, a CT Scan, Ultrasound, upper gastrointestinal series, and barium enema may be considered. When the injury is diagnosed by any of these studies, the injury should be repaired as soon as possible. It is important to keep in mind, that all traumatic diaphragmatic ruptures must be repaired at some point in time, no matter how large or small, or at what point in time they are discovered.

The exact mechanism of the rupture of the diaphragm is not known. The fusion lines of individual leaflets during the development of the diaphragm have been considered weak points that are predisposed to rupture. Surgery occurs more frequently in the left hemidiaphragm since the liver acts as a buffer, protecting the right hemidiaphragm. Research literature shows that the left hemidiaphragm rupture is as high as 85% in comparison to the right diaphragmatic rupture which is less than 15%. Although there is little mortality associated with the repair of the diaphragm, the morbidity associated with unrepaired lesions is considered significant. High mortality is associated with herniation of the diaphragm, or colon, and is directly related to the enteric contents entering into the pleural space.

Diaphragmatic rupture may be associated with major orthopedic injuries such as unstable pelvis, head injury, pulmonary contusions and myocardial contusions. These injuries would indicate the mechanism of injury, i.e., a sudden rise of intra-abdominal pressure created during the traumatic impact to the abdomen that is transmitted to the diaphragm. Hemodynamic instability secondary to hemorrhage from the liver or rib fracture would be an indication of a life threatening diaphragmatic rupture. Infection in trauma patients may represent a serious problem. Factors influencing the incidence of infection vary. Increased bacterial contamination in the field or from in-hospital patient care, blood transfusions, duration of the mechanical ventilation and the need for tracheotomy, severity of the injury should be considered.

A high injury severity score (ISS), pulmonary contusion, the presence of intravenous catheters, hypertension and increased bacterial contamination may contribute to the outcome of this injury.

The clinical manifestations of diaphragmatic injury, are generally related to concomitant injuries to adjacent organs. Patients with diaphragmatic rupture often have herniation of the abdominal viscera into the pleural space and may complain of shortness of breath, or present symptoms that are related with gastrointestinal obstruction when some type of abdominal viscera strangulation occurs. On physical examination, breath sounds are paramount, and they may be absent on the side of the herniation, and bowel sounds may be heard over the chest wall.

Patients in whom a diaphragmatic rupture is suspected, should have a naso-gastric tube inserted. Herniation of the stomach can be diagnosed on the chest roentgenogram if the tube appears to coil upward from beneath the diaphragm into the suspected area where the opening has occurred.

The nursing care of these patients begins as they enter the trauma admitting area or the Emergency Department. Here, a specific and well-rehearsed protocol for resuscitation is initiated. An immediate decision is made concerning the airway, and whether an endotracheal intubation should be performed. Estimation of volume status is the second most important factor. Evaluation of intravascular volume is performed by assessing the pulse for rate, rhythm and character and monitoring the patient's urinary output. Simultaneously, general perfusion of the skin and mental status should be assessed. The aggressiveness of the resuscitation depends on the mechanism of injury, the initial vital signs and the number of obviously injured organ systems. As previously mentioned, the diagnosis of a diaphragmatic tear is difficult because trauma to the diaphragm usually means multi-organ involvement. With gross herniation of visceral contents into the thoracic cavity, A mediastinal shift may occur resulting in respiratory distress and hemodynamic instability. The age of the patient and the quality of pre-hospital care is important data to be considered. The general protocol for blunt trauma includes assessment of airway, volume, and monitoring of vital signs. Lateral cervical spine, chest, and pelvic films should then be performed. A peritoneal tap as well as other additional radiological studies may include CAT scans and arteriograms. Nursing care in this acute phase aimed at assessment function and monitoring for cardiorespiratory deterioration. All procedures, such as placement of intravenous lines, arterial lines, peritoneal lavage, placement of central venous pressure lines, and insertion of Foley catheters, are preceded by the appropriate preparation including anesthesia. Aseptic conditions should be maintained for all invasive procedures. As the resuscitation proceeds and diagnostic information becomes available, appropriate specialists are notified and priorities are set. If necessary, surgery is non-scheduled and immediate. The role of the trauma nurses during the immediate postoperative phase remains crucial. Data obtained from physiologic monitoring, together with the clinical picture of the patient, identifies trends from which to develop a plan of care. In cooperation with the surgeon, continuous assessment of the patient's hemodynamic stability remains a priority. While in the Intensive Care Unit, most nursing diagnosis will be physiological as the patient's body attempts to adapt to the stress of surgery. This is why it is important to understand the mechanism of the injury and the pathophysiological consequences of the operative procedure.

Complications of the diaphragmatic rupture may result from the severity of the rupture, fluid overload, multiple blood transfusions, infection, or pre-existing medical condition. Nursing intervention is aimed at actual problems, or the prevention of these potential complications.

The management of a patient with diaphragmatic repair includes a nursing diagnosis of potential respiratory insufficiency due to possible paralysis of the repaired diaphragm. Good pulmonary care is dependent upon the amount of fluid infused during resuscitation and other sustained repaired injuries. The weaning strategies must be incorporated into the plan of care when attempting to extubate the patient with the diaphragmatic rupture repair along with protocols for suctioning. Identification of patient care activities that predispose a patient to fatigue is necessary since weaning requires muscle strength. Currently, the clinical bedside assessment tools that reflect tired or weak diaphragm are spirometric measurements used to evaluate wean readiness. In addition, chest roentgenograms are essential to determine the presence of pneumothorax or hemothorax and must be correlated with the auscultation of the lungs. The presence of enteric contents into the chest requires administration of intravenous antibiotics. The nasogastric tube placed in the Emergency Room may still be needed for stomach decompression.

Pain control in the postoperative phase a very high priority. Pain may be associated with the injury repair, or result directly from the injury. Frequent evaluation of pain medication is necessary, and appropriate narcotics and sedation should be ordered. Sedation often inhibits cough therefore, increasing the risk of atelectasis or pneumonia. In addition, high doses of morphine have been linked to the occurrence of cholecystitis in trauma patients. Although the focus of this critical phase remains the physiological response, the psychosocial assessment of the patient is equally important. Because trauma patients are not planned admissions, it is essential for the nurse to identify and evaluate family dynamics, stress, level of coping and the patient's motivational level. A continuous assessment will enable the nurse to plan interventions to help the patient to deal with this injury more effectively. Trauma patient's emotional status fluctuates, as adjustments to the injuries occur. Once the initial crisis of possible loss of life is realized, the individual must attempt to move on towards the rehabilitative phase. In order to decrease the length of hospital stays for patients presenting with the diaphragmatic rupture, it is important for nursing to focus in on specific nursing diagnosis that will enhance direct patient care. Ineffective breathing pattern related to possible paralysis of the diaphragm represents such nursing diagnosis.

Management considerations would be patient positions, results of postoperative chest roentgenograms to rule out hemothorax or pneumothorax and other ventilatory support nursing measures. Secondary complications relating to ineffective breathing pattern may be atelectasis, pneumonia, pulmonary infiltrates, and pleural effusions. Impaired gas exchange related to capillary membrane changes could result in being reduced by a balancing fluid management, intubation and ventilation, aggressive pulmonary toilet, and prevention of aspiration. The outcome of traumatic diaphragmatic rupture is related to complications and quality of nursing care. This is one of the most paramount issues one may focus upon when discussing the possibility that nursing may impact on the length of stay and the overall quality of patient care. Consistent with many trauma patients, the alteration of comfort and pain should be diagnosed by nursing. Ineffective breathing patterns due to pain secondary to the incision, rib fractures, and chest tubes may be a new experience for many patients following traumatic diaphragmatic rupture.

Pain control is a consideration consistent with the assessment phase. Patients receiving narcotics, either IV or through patient-controlled analgesia (PCA), pump, may be provided with sufficient or insufficient narcotics based on the patient's incision line, multiple system involvement, or a past history of drug involvement. Pain control for trauma patients may involve epidural and intercostal nerve blocks which can be both beneficial in pain relief, and improving upon a previous ineffective breathing pattern. Ventilator weaning, management of the chest tubes, and adequate ventilation must be considered overall when nursing evaluates an airway for breathing patterns.

Additional nursing diagnoses for the patient with diaphragmatic injury may be an actual potential for infection. This may be related to retained secretions, alteration of skin and musculoskeletal systems, and the chest tube insertion and incision. All trauma patients have an increased risk of potential infection resulting in pneumonia, empyema, or lung abscesses. Long-term care should be thought of upon admission of the trauma patient. Impaired gas exchange from atelectasis and retained secretion or secondary to immobility from injury, possible pulmonary emboli or ARDS should be also considered. Atelectasis and copious secretions may require drainage and/or physiotherapy.

The outcome of a diaphragmatic rupture varies and depends upon the magnitude of severity of injury, including multiple system injuries. Certainly, a patient with single system injury with a small diaphragmatic rupture has a better chance for a good outcome as compared to one who experienced a head injury, emergency thoracotomy, a laparotomy, and multiple long bone fractures.

SUGGESTED READING

1. S.M. Budassi: Trauma Notebook: Chest Trauma. *Journal of Emergency Nursing* 9(6):356-360;1982.
2. S.M. Burns: Preventing diaphragm fatigue in the ventilated patient. *Dimensions of Critical Care Nursing* 10(1):13-19;1991.
3. A.C. Cernaianu, W.A. Baldino: Esophageal and diaphragmatic injuries. *Topics in Emergency Medicine* 12(1):53-57;1990.
4. A.C. Cernaianu, A.J. DelRossi: Traumatic rupture of the diaphragm. *Trauma Quarterly* 6(3):53-63;1990.

5. R. Gelman: Diaphragmatic rupture due to blunt trauma: sensitivity of plain chest radiographs. *AJR* 156(51):51-57;1991.
6. K.L. Mattox, M.K. Allen: Emergency department treatment of chest injuries. *Emergency medicine clinics of north america* 2(4):783-798;1984.

NURSING RESEARCH: THE KEY TO EXCELLENCE IN NURSING PRACTICE

Elizabeth H. Winslow, PhD, R.N.

The University of Texas at Arlington
School of Nursing
Arlington, Texas

Florence Nightingale gave nursing research a brilliant start but, after her death, nursing research lost its focus and relevance. Nursing research has recently emerged as a viable, clinically applicable force which is having a powerful impact on how we practice and becoming the key to improving nursing practice and patient outcomes.

Nightingale, an astute observer who kept detailed records, is considered our first nurse researcher. During the Crimean War, Nightingale quickly identified major factors affecting mortality and morbidity among the soldiers and controlled those factors. She recognized that most of the soldiers were not dying from war wounds, but from infection, exposure, malnutrition, and dehydration. She instituted major sanitary reforms despite being hampered, at every step, by military authorities who resisted any change. When Nightingale arrived at Scutari, the main British hospital in the Crimean War, the mortality rate was 43%; 6 months later it was 2%.[1] After returning to England, Nightingale persuaded powerful friends to present her findings in Parliament using sophisticated statistics and pie charts she provided. Nightingale's findings triggered widespread reforms in the care of both military and civilian populations.

After Nightingale, nursing research entered what can be called the "Dark Ages of Nursing Research". Little nursing research was conducted and the research that was done focused on the nurse, the equipment, or modes of delivering care and not on the patient or the effects of nursing care. In a 1956 editorial in *Nursing Research*, Virginia Henderson asked why we were studying ourselves rather than studying patients and the practice of nursing: "If research in any occupation were divided into two categories: 1) studies of the workers, and 2)

Cardiac Surgery: Current Issues, Edited by A.C. Cernaianu and A.J. DelRossi Plenum Press, New York, 1992

studies of their work, which type would usually predominate? Would we find more research on lawyers or the law; on engineers or engineering; on cleaners or cleaning? In all these occupations ... the conclusion is the same - that there has been more research on practice than on the practitioner."[2] Henderson then posed the pivotal question: "Why is it then, that in our field, studies on the nurse outnumber studies on the practice of nursing more than ten to one?"

Henderson realized that clinical, patient-focused research was critical for providing a scientific basis for our practice and for improving our nursing care. Nurse-focused research would have only an indirect effect on practice. Despite Henderson's compelling comments, it was not until the 1970's that widespread clinical nursing research focusing on the content of our care was initiated. Now, abundant and clinically relevant nursing research exists to help enhance our care and improve patient outcomes. We need to read and use nursing research if we are to provide optimal patient care.

Numerous well designed and carefully executed nursing research studies have been conducted and the findings have been substantiated in replication and extension studies. The greater the extent our nursing practice is based on these and other studies, the higher the quality our nursing care will become. Below are several examples of nursing research we can and should be using.

SENSORY PREPARATION FOR PAINFUL PROCEDURES

Jean Johnson extensively studied how to best prepare patients for painful procedures.[3,4] She found that it was important to tell patients what to expect, but to tell them from their point of view describing what the patient would see, hear, feel and smell, rather than describing what would be done from the nurse's or physician's perspective. Johnson found that giving patients sensory information led to significant reductions in their distress and anxiety during procedures. Johnson's findings have been substantiated in a variety of subjects and settings.

When we are preparing patients for a procedure we need to tell them the most common sensations associated with the procedure. For example, if patients are to have cardiac catheterization, it is important that they be forewarned about the hot feeling associated with the dye injection. Then, when they suddenly feel as if they are on fire, they will realize that this is a normal, expected, and transient response and will not become anxious and upset. Johnson's research has had a dramatic effect on human suffering and can benefit millions of patients each day.

DECREASING DISCOMFORT ASSOCIATED WITH IM INJECTIONS

As nurses, we may give ten or more intramuscular injections each shift. How can we decrease the discomfort associated with these injections? Kruszewski and colleagues,[5] Rettig and Southby,[6] and other investigators have shown discomfort is decreased if the injection is given into a relaxed muscle. For example, when giving a dorsogluteal injection, ask the patient to "toe in"; this relaxes the gluteus and decreases injection pain. For injections in other sites, also position the patient to "soften" the muscle site and you'll soon be known for your ability to give an almost painless injection.

ORAL TEMPERATURES AND NASAL OXYGEN

We do not need to remove nasal oxygen in order to obtain an accurate oral temperature. In fact, by removing needed oxygen, we can jeopardize the patient's oxygenation status. A number of nurse researchers have shown that the tongue acts as an effective insulator and protects the thermometer from the effects of the air current.[7,8] This is good news for both nurses and patients because few people like rectal temperatures.

BEDPAN USE AND ABUSE

Good news surrounds another "sacred cow" - the bedpan. Winslow and colleagues measured oxygen consumption and cardiovascular response in 95 subjects.[9] They found that based on energy cost and cardiovascular parameters, there is little rationale for keeping patients in bed for toileting. In addition, multiple physiological and psychological benefits are associated with getting out of bed and the subjects overwhelmingly preferred out-of-bed toileting. The few other studies on toileting show similar results.

PREOPERATIVE TEACHING

Nursing research has shown the value of structured preoperative teaching.[10,11] Preoperative teaching decreases length of stay, complications, pain, and time to return to normal activities, and increases patient satisfaction. What is it about preoperative teaching that brings about these wonderful results? We teach surgical patients: 1) information - where they will go, when, where the incision will be, what tubes they will have, what NPO means, what they will feel, hear and see, etc; 2) skills - how to deep breathe, cough, turn, and get out of bed; and we give patients 3) psychological support and reassurance. All three components of preoperative teaching are important and the benefits of the teaching are reduced if any of these components is missing. Research has also shown that personal contact and individualization are essential. Audiovisual aids are useful, but cannot replace the human contact.

OXYGENATING PATIENTS BEFORE AND AFTER ENDOTRACHEAL SUCTIONING

Endotracheal suctioning (ETS), a routine nursing intervention, removes secretions, enhances airway patency, and promotes oxygenation. However, ETS also temporarily reduces oxygenation by interrupting oxygen supply while increasing oxygen need. Thus, suction-induced hypoxemia is a common and serious complication associated with ETS. Over 30 years of nursing research have clearly shown that hyperoxygenation before, during, and/or after ETS minimizes suction-induced hypoxemia.[12,13] Thus, every nurse should use some form of hyperoxygenation when suctioning critically ill patients to reduce the harmful effects of suctioning. Research also has shown that using the ventilator for hyperoxygenation is more effective than the manual resuscitation bag in minimizing suction-induced hypoxemia and untoward hemodynamic changes.[14]

USING SALINE RATHER THAN DILUTE HEPARIN TO FLUSH HEPARIN LOCKS IN ADULTS

Traditionally, dilute heparin has been used to flush and maintain the patency of peripheral intravenous infusion devices (IID), commonly referred to as heparin locks. However, heparin is expensive, and it is incompatible with multiple drugs;in addition, heparin causes heparin-induced thrombocytopenia and thrombosis, a rare but serious complication.[15] Since extremely small doses of heparin are effective in maintaining IID patency, many clinicians questioned whether heparin was even needed. This question led to numerous studies comparing the efficacy of sodium chloride and dilute heparin for maintaining IIDs in adults. In Epperson's classic study in 1984, no significant difference was found in IID patency when a heparin flush was compared with a saline flush solution.[16] Multiple, well designed studies since then have confirmed Epperson's findings.[17,18] Given the risks of heparin administration and the abundant research showing that a saline flush solution is as effective as dilute heparin in maintaining IID patency, it is time to routinely use a saline flush solution for IIDs in adults. Using heparin flush for heparin locks is an "outmoded, expensive, and potentially harmful procedure" - it is time to remove this procedure from our practice.[19]

CONCLUSIONS

We cannot be blind to the value and relevance of nursing research. We must read, share, and apply nursing research. This is not an option, but an obligation to our patients, ourselves, and our profession.

REFERENCES

1. I.B. Cohen: Florence Nightingale. *Scientific American* 250:128-137;1984.
2. V. Henderson: Research in nursing practice - When? *Nursing Research* 4:2;1956.
3. J.E. Johnson: Effects of structuring patient's expectations on their reactions to threatening events. *Nursing Research* 21:499-504;1972.
4. N.G. McHugh, N.J. Christman, J.E. Johnson: Preparatory information: What helps and why. *Am J Nursing* 82:780-782;1982.
5. A.Z. Kruszewski, S.H. Lang, J.E. Johnson: Effect of positioning on discomfort from intramuscular injections in the dorsogluteal site. *Nursing Research* 28:103-105;1979.
6. F.M. Rettig, J.R. Southby: Using different body positions to reduce discomfort from dorsogluteal injection. *Nursing Research* 31:219-221;1982.
7. F. Lim-Levy: The effect of oxygen inhalation on oral temperature. *Nursing Research* 31:150-152;1982.
8. A.J. Longman, J.A. Verran, J. Ayoub, J. Neff, A. Noyes: Research utilization: An evaluation and critique of research related to oral temperature measurement. *Applied Nursing Research* 3(1):14-19;1990.
9. E.H. Winslow, L.D. Lane, F.A. Gaffney: Oxygen uptake and cardiovascular response in patients and normal adults during in-bed and out-of-bed toileting. *J Cardiac Rehab* 4:348-354;1984.
10. E.C. Devine, T.D. Cook: A meta-analytic analysis of effects of psychoeducational interventions on length of postsurgical hospital stay. *Nursing Research* 32:267-274;1983.
11. D. Hathaway: Effect of preoperative instruction on postoperative outcomes: A meta-analysis. *Nursing Research* 35:269-275;1986.
12. C.A. Barnes, K.T. Kirchhoff: Minimizing hypoxemia due to endotracheal suctioning: A review of the literature. *Heart & Lung*, 15:164-176;1986.
13. K.S. Stone, B. Turner: Endotracheal suctioning - In *Annual Review of Nursing Research* Edited by J.J. Fitzpatrick, R.L. Taunton, J.Q. Benoliel; Springer, New York p 27-49;1989.
14. K.S. Stone: Ventilator versus manual resuscitation bag as the method of delivering hyperoxygenation before endotracheal suctioning. *AACN Clinical Issues* 1(2):289-299;1990.
15. P.A. Kuhar, K.M. Hill: White clot syndrome: When heparin goes haywire. *Am J Nurs* 91:626-629;1984.
16. E. Epperson: Efficacy of 0.9% sodium chloride injection with and without heparin for maintaining indwelling intermittent injection sites. *Clinical Pharmacy* 3:626-629;1984.
17. C.J. Goode, M. Titler, B. Rakel, D.S. Ones, C. Kleiber, S. Small, P.K. Triolo: A meta-analysis of effects of heparin flush and saline flush: Quality and cost implications. *Nursing Research* 40(6):324-330;1991.
18. F.Y. Peterson, K.T. Kirchhoff: Analysis of the research about heparinized versus non-heparinized intravascular lines. *Heart & Lung* 20(6):631-642;1991.
19. F.S. Downs: Editorial: How to make a difference. *Nursing Research* 40(6):323;1991.

CONTRIBUTORS

Steven F. Bolling, M.D.
Assistant Professor of Surgery
University of Michigan Hospitals
Ann Arbor, MI

Edward L. Bove, M.D.
Professor of Pediatric Cardiac Surgery
University of Michigan Hospitals
Ann Arbor, MI

Louis Brownstein B.A., C.C.P.
Department of Surgery, Division of Cardiothoracic Surgery
UMDNJ-Robert Wood Johnson Medical School at Camden
Director School of Cardiovascular Perfusion
Cooper Hospital/University Medical Center
Camden, NJ

Louis A. Brunsting, M.D.
Assistant Professor of Surgery
University of Michigan Hospitals
Ann Arbor, MI

Aurel C. Cernaianu, M.D.
Assistant Professor of Surgery
UMDNJ-Robert Wood Johnson Medical School at Camden
Director, Research Programs
Division of Cardiothoracic Surgery
Cooper Hospital/University Medical Center
Camden, NJ

Denton A. Cooley, M.D.
Professor of Clinical Surgery
University of Texas Medical School
Chief Surgeon
Texas Heart Institute
Houston, TX

G. Michael Deeb, M.D.
Associate Professor of Surgery
University of Michigan Hospitals
Ann Arbor, MI

Robert Fietsam, Jr., M.D.
Research Associate
Department of Surgery, Division of Cardiothoracic Surgery
Wayne State University School of Medicine
Detroit, MI

F. Mark Lupinetti, M.D.
Assistant Professor of Surgery
University of Michigan Hospitals
Ann Arbor, MI

Mark B. Orringer, M.D.
Professor and Head, Section of
Thoracic Surgery
University of Michigan Hospitals
Ann Arbor, MI

Anthony J. DelRossi, M.D.
Associate Professor of Surgery
UMDNJ-Robert Wood Johnson Medical School at Camden
Chairman, Department of Surgery
Head, Division of Cardiothoracic Surgery
Cooper Hospital/University Medical Center
Camden, NJ

Susan Kiley Eckert, MSN, R.N., CCRN
Administrative Director, Shock Trauma
Washington Hospital Center
Washington, DC

Jill Fikkert, BSN, R.N.
Visiting Nurses of So. Central Connecticut
New Haven, CT

T. James Gallagher, M.D.
Professor of Anesthesiology and Surgery
University of Florida College of Medicine
Chief, Critical Care Medicine
Shands Hospital
Gainesville, FL

Elizabeth Hahn Winslow, Ph.D., R.N.
Associate Professor
The University of Texas at Arlington
Arlington, TX
Research Consultant
Harris Methodist
Ft. Worth, TX

Gail Kaempf, MSN, R.N.
Perioperative Clinical Nurse Specialist
Presbyterian Medical Center of Philadelphia
Philadelphia, PA

Mark Kurusz, B.A., CCP
Chief Perfusionist
The University of Texas Medical Branch at Galveston
Galveston, TX

Joan Perks, MSN, R.N.
Manager of Emergency Services
Atlantic City Medical Center
1925 Pacific Avenue
Atlantic City, NJ

James R. Pluth, M.D.
Professor of Surgery
Mayo Medical School
Consultant, Thoracic and Cardiothoracic Surgery
Mayo Clinic-Scottsdale
Scottsdale, AZ

Bonnie Sakallaris, MSN, R.N., CCRN
Clinical Nurse Specialist
Washington Hospital Center
Washington, DC

Jeffrey P. Sites, BS, C.T., CCP
Cardiovascular and Extracorporeal Technologies
Plymouth, MN

Richard K. Spence, M.D.
Associate Professor of Surgery
UMDNJ-Robert Wood Johnson Medical School at Camden
Head, Section of General Vascular Surgery
Cooper Hospital/University Medical Center
Camden, NJ

Larry W. Stephenson, M.D.
Professor of Surgery
Chief, Division of Cardiothoracic Surgery
Wayne State University School of Medicine
Detroit, MI

Roger A. Vertrees, BA, CCP
Program Director
School of Cardiovascular Perfusion
Cooper Hospital/University Medical Center
Camden, NJ

Rosemary Volosin, R.N., MSN
Clinical Nurse Specialist
Division of Cardiothoracic Surgery
UMDNJ-Robert Wood Johnson Medical School at Camden
Cooper Hospital/University Medical Center
Camden, NJ

INDEX

Acidosis, 66, 67, 69, 70, 120, 122, 125, 176, 177, 179
ACT, 92, 96, 110, 131, 155
Adenosine phosphate, 110
Aggregation, 103, 169
AIDS, 91, 199
Albumin, 98, 100, 102, 169, 172
Aldosterone, 179
Alfentanil, 66
Alkalosis, 69
Alveolar ventilation, 65, 165
Aneurysm
  repair, 10, 16, 30, 76, 78, 79, 88, 89
  aneurysmectomy, 6, 26, 89, 184
Angina
  pectoris, 10, 26, 57, 144
  unstable preoperative, 46, 47, 94, 105, 112, 184, 187, 191
Annuloplasty, 5, 6, 56, 135
  bicommissural, 56
  Carpentier ring, 56
  size, 4, 5
Annulus, 6
Antiarrhythmic therapy, 183
Anticoagulation, 4, 58, 78, 87, 95, 111, 131, 133, 134, 149, 155, 163, 181, 182
  complications, 3
Antidiuretic, 96, 179
Antithymic Globulin (ATGAM), 36
Aorta
  aneurysms, 78, 79
  compliance, 105
  valve prosthesis type, 58
  valve stenosis, 57
  valvular insufficiency, 79
Apnea, 64
Aprotinin, 96, 98, 99
Arrhythmia, 16, 50, 119, 184
Aspirin, 96
Atelectasis, 179, 180, 186, 193, 194
Atheroembolization, 48
Atrial fibrillation, 81, 119, 187
Autograft, 10
Autologous
  donors, 93
  platelet-rich plasma, 98
  predonation, 92, 93

Autologous (*cont'd*)
  program, 93
Automatic implantable cardioverter, 184
Autonomic nervous system, 109, 110, 121
Autoregulation, 66, 113, 115
Autotransfusion, 95, 98, 100
  techniques, 95
Azathioprine, 36

Balloon septostomy, 83
Barbiturates, 64
Baroreceptor reflexes, 110
Benzodiazapines, 123
Biocompatibility, 167, 171
Biomaterials, 9, 161, 162, 165, 167–169, 173
Bioprostheses, 2–4, 78, 131
Blood
  compatibility, 161, 162
  flow velocity, 103, 104
  osmolality, 111
Bloodless cardiac surgery, 91, 92, 99
Bohr's effect, 112
Bovine pericardium, 77
Bridge to transplantation, 86
Bronchiectasis, 37
Bubble oxygenator, 147, 163, 164
Bypass
  partial, 153

Calcification, 2, 78, 131, 134
Calcium turnover, 2
Cardiac
  arrest, 81, 176, 178, 183, 184
  assist, 3, 18, 24, 25, 27–31, 87
  augmentation, 10, 11, 15, 17, 24
  catheterizations, 143
  contractility, 64, 66, 70
  failure models, 14
  filling pressures, 69
  index, 4, 57, 68, 176, 178, 180
  output, 14–16, 23, 56, 64–67, 69, 70, 103, 119, 120
  penetrating injury, 10
  transplantation, 9, 39, 40, 85–88, 91, 150
  valve surgery, 48, 60

Cardiomyopathy, 15–17, 25, 29, 30, 38, 52, 54
  dilated, 15–17, 25, 29, 30
Cardiomyoplasty, 9, 10, 14–17, 24, 25, 27, 29–31
  indications for, 16
  substitution, 16
Cardioplegia, 6, 33, 56, 57, 97, 99, 118, 152, 175
  cold blood, 57
  cold chemical, 118
  cold potassium, 57
Cardioversion, 176
Cardioverter defibrillator, 9, 183, 184
Carotid
  asymptomatic disease, 45, 48, 60
  bruit, 45
Catecholamines, 119, 121, 179
  endogenous, 121
Central nervous system, 131
Cerebral infarction, 44, 48, 59, 112, 113, 116, 118, 134, 135, 156, 176, 180
Chagas myocarditis, 16
Chest tubes, 117, 119, 142, 153, 182, 194
Chordae tendineae, 7, 8, 78, 89, 127
Circulatory arrest, 79, 80, 82
Class-1 antigens, 34, 35
Class-2 antigens, 34, 36
Coagulation
  coagulopathy, 9, 178
  factors, 95, 97, 98, 118, 154, 162, 168
Colloid, 94, 97, 180
Color Doppler, 50, 56, 60
Combined coronary and cerebrovascular disease, 43–49, 56–61, 64, 67, 95, 121, 123, 149, 164, 177
Commissural plication, 78
Commissurotomy, 6, 8, 135
Complete revascularization, 33, 35, 56, 90, 141
Compliance, 105, 106, 109, 114, 134, 183
  arteries, 109
Conditioning, 13–15, 18, 28, 29
Conduction system, 80
  disturbances, 119, 120
Conduit, 82, 85, 90, 144, 182
Congenital disease, 36
Congestive heart failure, 9, 24, 30
Contractility, 13–16, 64–66, 70
  forces, 77
  power, 9, 10
Conversion, 13, 186
Coumadin, 4
Counterpulsation, 20, 21, 31, 57
Cryoablation, 81, 184
Cryoprecipitate, 96
Crystalloid, 94, 95, 97, 178, 180
Current counter shock, 185
Cyclosporine, 34, 36, 39, 40, 85
Cystic fibrosis, 37, 147
Cytomegalovirus, 91

Dacron fabric, 77
DDAVP, 96, 98
Defibrillation, 175, 185–187
  thresholds, 186
Defibrillator, 9, 140, 142, 183–185, 187
Defibrination, 168
Desensitizing, 118
Desmopressin, 96
Dextran, 95
Diaphragm
  hernia, 149, 160
  traumatic rupture, 188, 194
Diffusion, 65, 66, 101, 102, 106–108, 111, 112, 114, 164, 165, 167, 168, 172
  mechanism, 102
Dimethylsiloxane, 166, 171
Dissection, 79, 81, 94, 140–142, 181
Disseminated intravascular coagulation, 121
Donor organs, 39
Doppler examination, 52
Dor, 89
Doxorubicin, 15, 29
Duramedic, 1
Dysrhythmias, 176, 177

Edema, 95, 106, 134, 176, 179
Eisenmenger's Syndrome, 37, 38
Ejection fraction, 4, 7, 14–17, 33, 49, 54, 60, 73, 104, 105
EKG, 38, 117, 119–121, 182
Elastance, 15
Electrocortical depression, 113
Emboli, 135, 180, 194
Embolic-free survivorship, 7
Emphysema, 38
Endarterectomy, 43–48, 59, 60
Endoaneurysmorrhaphy, 77, 78, 88
Endocardial
  biopsy, 33
  mapping, 184
  resection, 184
Endotak, 185
Endothelial cells, 34, 109
Endotracheal tube, 123, 153
Enzyme, 12, 27, 63, 117
  induction, 63
Eosinophilic granulomatosis, 37
Erdheim's cystic medionecrosis, 79
Erythropoietin, 93, 98, 99
Etomidate, 64
Extra-cranial revascularization, 43
Extracorporeal
  centrifugal blood pump, 86
  oxygenation, 147, 158, 173

Factor VIII, 96
Fahreus-Linqvist factor, 111

Fast-twitch, 11
Fatigue resistance, 12, 13, 28
Fentanyl, 66
Ferropyrolite, 1
Fibrillation, 14, 81, 118, 119, 124, 141, 142, 184–187
Fibrin, 96, 97
Fibrin glue, 96, 97
Fibrinogen, 96, 102
Fibroblasts, 34
Flexible ring, 6
Flow
  disturbance, 109
  laminar flow, 104–106, 109, 112, 133, 162
  rates, 112–114, 116, 178
  velocities, 109
Fluid transport system, 108, 109
Fluorocarbon, 170
Fluosol, 97, 99
Flux rate, 171
Foley catheters, 117, 192
Forane, 65
Fresh frozen plasma, 96, 97, 141
Frictional forces, 108
Functional Class, 16, 17, 57

Gaseous microemboli, 44
Glenn shunt, 82
Globulins, 102
Glycogen, 120
Glycogenolysis, 179
Gradients, 1, 3, 4, 106, 121–124, 164, 165, 167
Grafts, 10, 14, 21, 72, 79, 89, 140–143, 181
  patency, 57
  ringed intraluminal, 89

Halothane, 65
Hancock, 1
Heart
  blocks, 134
  global failure, 14
  heart-lung transplantation, 33, 39, 40
  HeartMate, 86, 87
  transplant, indications for, 36
Heat, 112
Helper cell, 34–36
Hematocrit, 93, 94, 102, 112, 113, 121, 147
Hemodilution, 94, 95, 98, 99, 111, 112
  isovolemic, 94, 99
Hemoglobin, 66, 69, 91, 97–99, 112, 120, 156, 176
  fresh, 97, 98, 156
Hemolysis, 133, 147, 156
Hemophiliacs, 96
Hemopump, 86
Hemothorax, 193
Hepatitis, 91
Homografts, 79
Homologous transfusion, 92, 98
Hybrid, 170, 173
Hydrophobic, 166, 167
Hydrostatic pressure, 179
Hydroxyethyl starch, 95, 100
Hypercarbia, 119
Hypercoagulability, 162
Hyperglycemia, 111, 120, 177, 178
Hypertension, 37, 38, 50, 54, 64, 110, 117, 119, 149, 160, 177, 191
Hypocalcemia, 177
Hypoglycemia, 120
Hypokalemia, 177
Hyponatremia, 177
Hypothalamus, 110, 121
Hypothermia, 8, 66, 79, 80, 82, 95, 111–113, 116–121, 123–125, 175–178, 182
Hypovolemia, 119, 121, 123
Hypoxia, 119, 120, 153, 177, 187
Hysteresis effect, 105

Ileus, 120, 181, 182
IMA, 140–143, 181
Immune response, 34–36
Immunosuppression, 33, 40, 171
Immunotherapy, 35, 36
Infection, 9, 26, 36, 37, 39, 86, 91, 139, 140, 181, 182, 186, 187, 191, 193, 194, 197
  rates, 182
Inhalation, 65, 66, 123, 201
Inotropes, 38
Insulin, 37, 120, 124, 177–179
Intensive care unit, 68, 117, 122, 142, 187, 192
Intermediate ICU, 127
Internal mammary artery, 1, 44, 73, 79, 94, 102, 121, 140, 142, 153, 181
Intra-aortic balloon pump, 9, 46, 86, 157
Iron
  therapy, 93, 98
  anemia, 93
Ischemic heart disease, 10, 14, 16, 17, 38, 43–45, 50, 52, 54, 56, 61, 71, 72, 110, 130, 137
Isoforane, 65

Jehovah's Witness, 94, 99

Kallikrein, 96
Kent bundle, 81
Kinetic energy, 103, 106
Lactate, 68–70, 114
Lactic acidosis, 66, 67, 70
Latissimus dorsi, 9, 10, 13–18, 21, 23–25, 27–30
Law of Laplace, 107
Leucocyte, 121
Liver-spleen scan, 190
Lung
  hypoplasia, 149

Lung (*cont'd*)
  indications for transplant, 37
Lymphocytes, 34–36

Macrophages, 34, 35
Major histocompatibility antigens (MHC), 34
Malignant ventricular tachyarrhythmia, 183
McGoon repair, 5
Mechanical
  assist devices, 24
  prosthesis, 58, 78
  valves, 1, 3, 4, 58, 78, 133–135, 181
Mediastinal tumor, 164
Membrane oxygenator, 9, 13, 96, 102, 116, 145–149, 153–173, 178, 194
Metabolic
  acidosis, 67, 120, 176–177
  rate, 112, 115, 118, 120, 122
Metocurine iodine, 123
Microcirculation, 113, 179
Microcytic anemia, 93
Microemboli, 44, 65, 180
Midazolam, 64
Mitral valve
  annulus, 78
  dysfunction, 49, 52, 54
  excision of, 4, 5, 76–79, 88
  incompetence of ischemic origin, 54
  prolapse, 56
  regurgitation, 4, 5, 7, 49, 50, 52, 54, 56, 60, 61, 78, 127
  repair, 54, 61
  replacement, 1, 7, 54, 56, 60, 61, 78, 89, 131
Mock circulation device, 19, 20
Morbidity, 6, 45, 130, 131, 141, 191, 197
Morphine, 66, 123, 125, 193
Multiple organ failure, 13, 36, 67, 68, 72, 80, 81, 120, 147, 192, 194, 199, 200
Multivessel disease, 75
Murmur, holosystolic, 5
Murray's Law, 109
Muscle
  fatigue, 10, 11, 21
  fibrosis, 24
Myocardial
  augmentation, 8, 9
  contractility, 16
  damage, 131
  depression, 176
  fibrosis, 78
  infarction, 26, 56–60, 76, 78, 88, 96, 178, 184
  injuries, 57
  ischemia, 36, 49, 50, 54, 57, 70
  protection, 56, 57, 176
  reperfusion injury, 97
Myocardial (*cont'd*)
  revascularization, 45, 48, 49, 52, 54, 57–61, 99, 143
  tumors, 16
Myosin, 11, 12, 20, 27, 28

Narcotics, 63–66, 123, 193, 194
Nasogastric tubes, 120
Nerve stimulator, 12
Neurological deficits, 113
Neuromuscular impulses, 123
Nitrous oxide, 65, 66
Non-disabling strokes, 43
Non-pulsatile
  CPB, 44
  flow, 106, 179
Non-turbulent, 162
Normothermia, 69, 71, 88, 117, 118
Nursing
  care, 9, 125, 153, 180, 182–184, 192, 194, 197, 198
  research, 9, 197–201

Ohm's Law, 103
OKT3, 36
Omental flap, 34
Operative
  mortality, 17, 38, 39, 49, 54, 56
  risk, 48, 54, 56, 60, 75
Oxidative phosphorylation, 11–13
Oxygen
  carrying capacity (hemoglobin), 66, 69
  consumption, 13, 16, 17, 28, 66–70, 112, 114, 116, 119, 120, 175, 199
  demands, 66, 69, 118, 119
  extraction, 66–69
  transport, 56, 63, 70
Oxyhemoglobin, 69, 112, 120, 176
  dissociation curve, 69, 112, 176

Pacemaker, 15, 24, 89, 119, 140
Papillary muscle
  disruption, 5, 6
  dysfunction, 50, 54
  rupture, 52, 56
  scarring, 52
Patch
  lead, 185
  pericardial, 6
Pavulon, 123
PEEP, 38, 157, 180, 182
Pentastarch, 98, 100
Percutaneous transluminal coronary angioplasty, 75, 88, 146
Perfluorocarbon emulsions, 97
Perfluorodecalin, 170
Perioperative
  complications, 45
  stroke, 45, 48
Peripheral circulation, 56, 106
Permeability, 179

Pharmacologic support, 117, 123
Phlebotomy, 93, 98, 100
Physiologic dead space, 176
Plasma, 79, 95–100, 102, 103, 111, 121, 141, 156, 166–169, 179
Plasmin, 96
Platelet, 44, 95, 141, 147, 162, 169, 179
  dysfunction, 95–99, 121, 147, 169, 179
  microaggregation of, 44
Platelet-rich plasma, 95, 98, 99
Pneumothorax, 186, 193
Poiseuille's Law, 106, 108
Polyclonal antibodies, 36
Postoperative
  bleeding, 95, 142, 179
Potential energy, 103, 108
Precapillary sphincter muscle, 110
Preconditioning, 19, 20
Predictors of outcome, 49
Preservation, 4, 7, 33, 34, 89, 96, 113, 118, 131, 163
Pressure
  oncotic, 178
  osmotic, 94
Primary idiopathic bronchiolitis, 37
Primary pulmonary hypertension, 37, 38, 149
Propofol, 64
Propranolol, 14, 15, 23
Prostaglandins, 169
Protein denaturation, 166, 170
PTCA, 75, 76, 88, 138, 147
Pulmonary
  artery occlusion pressure (PAOP), 52, 134
  artery pressure, 14, 57, 134
  embolus, 37
  fibrosis, 38, 40
  hypertension, 37, 38, 50, 54, 149, 160
  system, 119, 177
Pulsatile
  circulation, 79
  flow, 105, 106, 114, 116, 179
  perfusion, 114, 163
  pump, 87, 105, 116
Pulseless perfusion, 113, 114

Reactive hyperemia, 35, 110
Regurgitation, 3–5, 7, 49, 50, 52, 54, 56, 60, 61, 78, 127, 128, 133
  bruit, 4–7, 15, 17, 24, 52, 76, 78, 82, 83, 89, 136, 190
Rejection, 9, 34, 36, 38–40, 86, 87
Renin, 179
Reoperation, 3, 4, 7, 49
Respiratory failure, 120, 147–150, 158
Restenosis, 75, 88, 181
Rewarming, 79, 117, 120–125, 141, 177, 178, 182
Reynold's number, 104, 105, 112, 113
Rheology, 101, 111, 114
Risk factors, 57, 61, 73, 114
Roller pump, 153, 154, 163
Ruptured tendineae, 5, 7, 136

Saphenous vein grafts, 72, 140
Screen oxygenator, 164
Segmental wall dysfunction, 54
Semi-organic polymers, 167
Sepsis, 67, 70, 149
Serine proteinase inhibitor, 96
Sheer stress, 108, 109, 112
Shivering, 66, 119–125, 176–178
Sinus bradycardia, 119
Skeletal muscle ventricules, 8–21, 24–32
Slow-twitch, 11
SMV, 9, 18–21, 23, 24
Sodium nitroprusside, 67
Sodium thiopental, 63, 64
Sternotomy, 94, 137, 140, 141, 186
Steroids, 36
Stroke
  risk, 43–45
  volume, 14, 16
  work index, 16
Stroma-free hemoglobin (SFH), 97
Subacute bacterial endocarditis, 6
  fibroelastosis, 85, 91
  viability index, 23
Sudden cardiac death, 183, 184
Sufentanil, 66
Supraventricular tachycardia, 81
Surface interaction, 24, 44
Surfactant, 170, 179
Sympathetic system, 110
Syncope, 80, 81, 183

Tachyarrhythmias, 81, 89
Tachycardia, 81, 119, 123, 125, 176, 183–188
Teflon, 171
Temperature gradients, 121, 124
Thermoreceptors, 121
Thermoregulation, 121, 122
Third space syndrome, 179
Thoracoscopy, 190
Thrombin, 96, 172
Thrombocytopenia, 169, 200
Thromboembolism, 1, 3, 78, 130, 131, 133–135
  complications, 3, 4, 21, 87
Thrombogenicity, 133, 168, 173
Thromboresistance, 162
Thrombosis, 1, 82, 130, 162, 186, 200
Tidal volume, 38, 65, 120
Tissue oxygenation, 110, 119
Transesophageal echocardiography (TEE), 52
Transfusion, 8, 70, 91, 92, 94–100, 163, 172
Transient ischemic attack (TIA), 45
Transplant, 8, 9, 25, 26, 31, 33–41, 85–88, 91, 145, 150, 163, 173
  great vessels, 82, 90

Trasylol, 96, 99
Tricuspid atresia, 82, 90
Trypsin deficiency, 37
Tubular
heat exchanger, 153, 155
necrosis, 96, 121
Turbulence, 104, 105, 112–115, 162
Turbulent flow, 104, 105, 112, 162

Ultrasound, 114, 115, 149, 190

Valium, 123
Valve
assessment, 5
ball-and-cage, 3, 4
Carpentier-Edwards, 1, 133
disease, 36, 52, 54, 56, 57, 61, 127
failure, 1, 2, 4
Ionescu-Shiley pericardial, 1
Medtronic-Hall, 1
Omni-Science, 1
replacement, 8, 1, 4, 7, 49, 54, 56–58, 60, 61, 78, 89, 99, 127, 128, 130, 131, 134, 135, 179, 181
St. Jude, 3, 1, 89, 131
Starr-Edwards, 1, 3, 7, 131
valve-anticoagulant group, 58
wear, 1
Valvuloplasty, 6–8, 78
Van't Holt effect, 175
Vasoactive, 111
Vasodilators, 123, 180
Vasopressin, 96
Vasopressors, 117
Vasospasm, 143, 182
Velocity, 14, 102–106, 108, 112, 115, 163
Ventricle
aneurysm, 16, 30, 76, 78, 88, 89
assist device, 86
contractility, 14
contractions, 119
dilatation, 54
dysfunction, 46, 49, 50, 52, 54, 78, 89, 138
fibrillation, 118, 119, 124, 142, 184–186
pacing, 15
right pressure, 14
septal defects, 85, 172
wall replacement, 14
Versed, 123
Viscosity, 69, 94, 102–104, 106, 108, 111–114, 118, 121, 162, 170, 176
Viscous
friction, 104, 108, 112
resistance, 102
vonWillebrand's Factor, 96

Wall motion score, 54, 61
Warfarin, 58, 87
Watershed infarctions, 44
Wolff-Parkinson-White syndrome, 90
Wrapping, technique for, 15

FSC
www.fsc.org
MIX
Papier | Fördert gute Waldnutzung
FSC® C083411

Zeitfracht Medien GmbH
Ferdinand-Jühlke-Straße 7
99095 Erfurt, Deutschland
produktsicherheit@kolibri360.de